A WAY OUT

DISEASE, DECEPTION, AND **THE TRUTH** ABOUT **HEALTH**

MATTHEW GRACE

This book is written as a source of information only. Matthew
Grace is not a medical doctor and does not prescribe medicine
and/or treatments for disease. This book is a study of The Laws
of Nature and is an attempt to remind the reader that health is
a natural birthright, simple, and attainable by all. The author
and the publisher disclaim any liability for any adverse effects
arising from the use or application of the information
contained herewith.

Published by Matthew Grace
matthewpgrace@hotmail.com
www.matthewgrace.com

This title is available for bulk purchase, special promotions
and premiums. For all domestic and foreign rights information
and sales, please contact

LifeTime Media Inc.

352 Seventh Avenue
New York, NY 10001
2 1 2 . 6 3 1 . 7 5 2 4

www.lifetimemedia.com
sales@lifetimemedia.com

To all the great and brave souls who have had
the courage to tell the truth in a world full of lies.

ACKNOWLEDGMENTS

...To great Nature who never stops teaching and reminding us of the miraculous universe in which we live.

...To my sister Nicole who's unconditional support, good humor, and appreciation are rare gifts that are immeasurable.

...To all those who lent their support when things got rough: Special thanks to Nicole and Bill Keck and Dafna Mordecai. Also thanks to: Doreen Casper, Louis Lanza, Sophie Biddle, Janna Copley, Barbara Hackett, Erica Burke, Carlos Aldebot (who always reminds me "what doesn't kill you makes you stronger"), Marcus Lovett, Gordon Elliot, Marianne Hettinger, Ann Barbour, Judy Dugan, Andrew Brooks, Richard Corman, Tom Dicillio, Wendi Singer Saggese, Isabelle Forte, and Rachel Lemanski.

...To my teachers Dr. John Tilden, Herbert Shelton, T.C. Fry, and Nature.

...To more of my friends: Kevin Moccia, Charles Ward, Blossom Blue Sky, Lori Evans, Nancy Wadsworth, Karen Ranzi, Bettina Belonde, Josephine Vinci, Tommy Tune, Cindy Joseph, Angela Fischetti Mickey Dissend, Aaron Gorbaty, Tatiana Kozlova, and to Rob Matsner for his generous donation and belief in this work.

...To those who had a hand in getting this book published: Vince Cordaro, Dr. Carlyn Cahill, Lisa Kindig, and John Grace. To Casey Stewart-Lindley, my editor (amongst other things) who worked enthusiastically and tirelessly to get this book ready. Your ability, tenacity and enthusiasm provided the last and oh so necessary push to get this book out. You are a true godsend. Thank you.

...To Mom and Dad, who have always done their best to support me. Thank you. Now, eat your fruit!

...To all the wonderful animals that teach me so much about presence, joy and unconditional love.

...To all my adversaries, inside and outside, a sincere Thank You.

Is an open mind a choice or an endowment? I used to think I knew. I don't. Is my mind open? I'm not sure but it feels like it is. I like that. Whatever force is responsible, Thank You, and I pray that the opening and broadening may go on as long as necessary.

PRAISE FOR A WAY OUT

Wow! A Way Out has forever changed my life and the way I view food and medicine. Matthew Grace is a genius and his book is full of insight and truth. Share this book with everyone; it will change the world!

—Rory Freedman

This book is a must for anyone who wants to overcome any and all disease and regain their natural birthright: health.

—Anonymous, New York, NY

Matthew Grace's journey is an incredible testament to the healing power of the body if you just give it the right tools.

—Chris Spartz

What an inspirational story and a wonderful book.

—Lynn C. Arnet

I just finished A Way Out and it is wonderful. It is articulate, informative, and to the point. Matthew speak[s] with devoted passion and a true desire to help others. I applaud this accomplishment and encourage the universe to have it reach MANY welcomed hearts and minds!

—Peter Humer

I can't tell you how much I enjoyed reading the book...[It] has forever changed me, and I will always be grateful.

—Phyllis Polito

C O N T E N T S

―――――◦◆◦―――――

INTRODUCTION

---- ❖ ◆ ❖ ----

The mind of man is taken far more with disguises than with realities.

—Ralph Waldo Emerson

Imagine being in a dark and crowded room. With every other step you smash your shin against a table, hit your head on a lamp, smack your hip on the corner of a desk, and repeatedly trip over pieces of furniture. Everyone around you is tripping and injuring him or herself as well. You make efforts to stop injuring yourself, but despite your good intentions you keep falling. There somebody who is giving out pills that will deaden the pain of your injuries; and the pills are very popular in the land of the dark, as everyone is suffering cuts and bruises.

A collective decision is made to raise money in hopes of figuring out how to make furniture that is not so dangerous, and to design clothing that will protect everyone from injury. The decision to name all the injuries suffered from particular falls and collisions is also agreed upon, including BHS (Bruised Hip Syndrome), TA (Twisted Ankleitis), and BHD (Bruised Head Disease). The acronyms are repeatedly used by physicians and the general population until they become part of the daily lexicon. Committees are formed, money is raised, celebrities (out of the goodness of their hearts) speak out in increased "awareness" until research begins to find the cures for these conditions. Experts suggest that walking faster will help, but more people end up getting injured. An expert from a top university claims that it must be some type of microbe, either a germ or a virus that causes people to bang into furniture. Another expert says his study reveals that walking backward is the answer; yet another claims the problem is instead a genetic predisposition and begins lobbying for additional funds for genetic research. The years go on and on, and despite billions of dollars spent on the research and the advice of highly educated men and women, people in the dark continue to trip and fall at an increasing rate. ***Lack of money or lack of proper treatments and "cures" is not the issue.***

As long as you are in the dark it really does not matter what you decide, how intent you are at not banging into furniture, how much research is done, or what experts say.

The only real solution is to turn on the light.

Our civilization is in the midst of a severe health crisis. We are stumbling in the dark, searching for solutions in places where they simply do not exist. We live in a world where few, if any, human beings die of natural causes. To die of natural causes, you must live a natural life. In today's modern culture, people live unnatural lives and, thus, die of unnatural causes. Most human beings succumb to heart disease and cancer treatments and die with debilitated and decrepit, disease-filled bodies, brittle and weakened bones, and failing organs. We stumble around in the dark, imagining that if we *"run faster,"* raise more money, and do more research, things may improve. This is our present plight, but it does not have to be so.

The following work is offered as a safe and tremendously effective option for those suffering from disease and physical discomfort, whether labeled incurable, chronic, or hereditary, and for those who simply want to live with optimum health.

My wish is that you read and re-read this book with *new ears*. It is not so much *if* you read this book but *how* you read this book. Please do not fall into the trap of "I've already heard that" or "Oh, that's just like what I learned at that seminar," etc. This is a horrible practice that disallows you to perceive what is really being said instead of your version or interpretation of what is being said. You may hear many words that you have heard before, but perhaps they may be saying something utterly different and altogether separate from what you may already know. Only an empty cup can be filled.

The general mass of our population is not exposed to thousands of recoveries that take place every year from *all* types of disease, whether deemed "incurable" or not. Those who *understand* the way the human body works and those who abide by these Laws of Nature invariably regain their health.

The aim of this work is to present you with knowledge that will enrich your life and is something that *really* works. These principles are not my ideas; they are the timeless, primordial and eternal Laws of Nature. Much like Newton, Copernicus, and Galileo represented and reported their observations of the natural world, this work is an attempt to describe what has been observed in nature without the distorting and tainted effects of opinion (it has been said that opinion exists between ignorance and knowledge) or "beliefs of the day." Whether you are suffering from what is called chronic, incurable, or terminal disease, or you just want to lose weight, look better, and feel better, these laws will provide you with the best opportunity to do just that, simply, inexpensively, and more effectively than anything else.

Years ago I was told that I had an "incurable" disease.

Wheelchair-bound, I was unable to move my legs, unable to stand or walk, constantly fatigued, and suffering severe numbness throughout my body. Doctors told me that I had multiple sclerosis and spinal cord degeneration. I was given no chance for recovery; a couple of the doctors sympathetically encouraged me to enroll in a handicapped employment service. I was told of the list of steroids and other drugs given to those in my condition. The doctors could not tell me what caused this disease, how to cure it, or say for sure if the drugs had any beneficial effects. Of course, all of the drugs prescribed had damaging effects, commonly called "side" effects. I, therefore, refused ALL of their treatments, as none of them made any sense.

THE IDEA THAT THERE IS SUCH A THING AS AN "INCURABLE DISEASE" IS SIMPLY NOT TRUE. DISEASE IS JUST THAT —DIS-EASE— OR LACK OF EASE IN THE BODY.

I am now back to a vigorous exercise regime that includes bicycle riding, yoga, rebounding (mini-trampoline), running, calisthenics, and weight training.

For the past fifteen years I have witnessed the powerful and immutable Laws of Nature restore health to sick and seemingly hopelessly ill people, whether they were diagnosed with cancer, "AIDS," tumors, arthritis, chronic digestive problems, obesity, hypoglycemia, or diabetes. Those who commit themselves and adhere to nature's wisdom return themselves to health.

Just as quickly as nature aids those who live in accordance with her laws, those who refuse to recognize these tenets suffer and are forced to exist in the confusion, darkness, and fear of our presently accepted notions of health and disease, habitually resorting to dangerous and often deadly drugging and invasive surgeries. Nature is unforgiving. No matter how accepted or revered our physicians and their treatments of the day may be, Natural Laws remain unaffected. *When you disregard Nature's Laws, it does not matter who is in agreement with you or what expert advice you are following. You will pay the price. No one, no matter how educated or respected, can fly a lead kite.*

The present paradigm for dealing with disease is failing miserably, while Nature's way continues to provide relief and healing to those who have sought out the truth and have been willing to make the necessary changes.

> *The major cause of your illness: you have forgotten your true nature.*
>
> —Boethius
> *Consolation of Philosophy*

Our "health experts" provide us with drug after drug and treatment after treatment, yet the health of our citizens continues to decline. Despite billions of dollars spent on thirty years of research and trillions of dollars on "treatments," more people today suffer from cancer than ever before and still no cure exists. At the same time the cancer rate continues to climb. No real solutions have been found, only an ever-increasing number of treatments. Cancer screening tests are often free or extremely cheap. The "treatments," however, are a different story.

Few, if any of us, understand a doctor's methods of diagnosis and ask nothing about the remedies dispensed. Despite our confusion, we assume that what we are being told is the truth and the most effective course of action in the treatment of our symptoms.

There are countless "health experts" on the scene with new protocols and treatments for the sick, all professing that they have the answers to treating disease. Year after year, new and exciting (often bizarre) techniques are introduced to an ignorant public who is promised "miracle cures" and "wonder drugs." Watch a newscast this evening and you have a good chance to hear about a "hopeful" new drug or medical "breakthrough."

Despite the continuous hype, nobody seems to recognize the emptiness of these promises or the continuing decline of our health. The confusion deepens with each passing fad and mania. True health remains a mystery to the masses.

Great truths do not take hold of the hearts of the masses.
— Chuang Tse

Why is it that health has become such a confusing issue? Has the creative force that put together this amazing universe made a mistake? Why is it that animals (in their pristine environment) do not live such diseased lives? There are no animals in nature with arthritis, asthma, cancer, obesity, heart disease, strokes, "AIDS," osteoporosis, the flu, etc. No animals in nature are injecting themselves with dangerous vaccines or flu shots. There are no animals taking supplements or protein powders or going on diets, eating according to their blood type, or weighing their food. They simply abide by their natural instincts and get along just fine.

Unfortunately, our natural instincts concerning nutrition are buried DEEP beneath the morass of misinformation and propaganda that exists in today's world. We are submerged in a sea of illusions and deceptions that are so rampant and persuasive that the truth is virtually out of our realm of consideration. The power of our natural intuition has been all but nullified by our "schooling" and the ubiquitous presence of big business. The medical lobby in Washington is second only to the oil lobby in its influence on lawmakers. Modern medicine's deluded misrepresentations concerning health and disease have so heavily indoctrinated our day-to-day thinking that an outside, objective observer would see little chance for most people to think clearly about these issues. The mental corruption runs so deep that there are only a small number of citizens that are even willing to listen to another point of view.

Our unconscious acceptance of such specious and misleading information from our "experts" is the reason why we are at the mercy of disease and powerless to question our doctors and their diagnosis of our illnesses and choice of treatments.

ARE HUMAN BODIES FLAWED?

Is there any reason why disease has become a part of our everyday life and accepted as natural? Did nature make some mistakes when designing the human body? Why are we the only species on the planet that suffer such disease-ridden lives? Alas, we are NOT the only species on the planet that suffer disease. Our house pets have also become obese and suffer from arthritis, upset stomachs, toothaches, cancer, and the rest of the gamut of pain that humans endure. What is the common denominator between our house pets and ourselves?

The glaring and most obvious factor is the quality of food that we and our house pets ingest. This food is of a completely different quality than what is ingested in nature.

Nature has provided EVERYTHING necessary for life: sunshine, air, water, and the necessary instincts to stay out

WE ARE THE ONLY SPECIES ON THE PLANET EATING COOKED, DEVITALIZED FOOD.

of harm's way. Nature has not forgotten anything. The complete recipe for our well-being and disease-free lives is at hand. The question must be asked. Why is it that we suffer so much disease?

PAIN IS THE GREATEST MESSENGER

Pain is always trying to get a message to us. It is an indication that something is amiss, and an adjustment must be made to return ourselves back to comfort. If the actions taken to remove the pain do not work or, worse, exacerbate the pain, it ought to be an indication that our efforts need to be re-examined. Our modern civilization is in a lot of pain. The methods presently practiced are increasing our pain, as more people are suffering disease than ever before. If we were truly serious about solving this problem, the answers could be found.

However, a major problem exists in our society. We are turned in to the QUICK-FIX mentality. We have a headache and want immediate relief and so reach for a painkiller or an aspirin. Our stomach is upset, so we take something to quell the symptom for instant relief. We are feeling empty so we overeat. Very rarely do we consider the message that is being sent to us by our bodies or spend a minute wondering over the possible CAUSE of our discomfort. Instead, we create a pattern of numbing and suppressing the body, which, in turn, creates a veritable gagging of Nature's communication with us. This impatient, automatic reaction to obtain relief is a major cause of our dire health crises.

IF YOUR WISH FOR RELIEF IS GREATER THAN YOUR WISH FOR UNDERSTANDING, YOU WILL GET NEITHER GENUINE RELIEF NOR GENUINE UNDERSTANDING.

Imagine a dammed lake that is being continuously flooded by an over-flowing river. The added pressure creates cracks in the wall of the dam. A messenger boy repeatedly rides into town to tell the leaders of the village that there are cracks in the dam. Instead of gathering some engineers and going to see for themselves in order to assess the damage and pinpoint the cause of cracks, the town leaders give the young boy some plaster and spackling tools and tell him to keep quiet about the news of the weakening dam so as not to upset the townspeople. The leaders, convinced by each other that they have done the right thing, go on about their business disregarding the imminent warnings. The young boy is able to do some temporary repairs. Cosmetically the dam appears to be fine, but appearances cannot fool the Laws of Nature. Disaster is imminent.

This is an example of foolish decision-makers disregarding signs of impending doom. Though deep down they sense the wrongness of it, they convince each other that sending the messenger boy to mend the cracks in the wall is a responsible and appropriate measure. Their nodding heads and collective agreements may provide a temporary and false feeling of comfort, but this charade will not affect the inevitable outcome.

Modern society does the same when dealing with disease. When any physical discomfort or distress appears, we take a pill to alleviate the pain; this quick and cosmetic approach *does nothing to remove the CAUSE of the pain*. However, the accepted and "normal" method of dealing with pain by getting rid of it is no different than the ignorant and dangerous act of silencing the messenger boy and sending him to spackle the wall of the collapsing dam.

QUICK-FIX SOLUTIONS LEAD TO LONG-TERM DISASTERS.

Not only does this method of suppressing symptoms negate the need for any understanding of the cause of pain, the substances that are used to mask the pain can cause many more bodily sufferings to come.

The insanity of this covering up and disregarding the body's message is dangerous enough, but if one takes the time to consider the very substances used for the masking, with all their inherent deleterious, disease producing effects, the madness of the whole process begins to reveal itself.

ALL drugs and pharmaceutical products have what the

doctors and drug companies call "side effects," which are debilitating symptoms caused by the very substance that is supposed to be making us well. These "side effects" may include everything from headaches, vomiting, and fevers to kidney failure, heart failure, and that annoying little "SIDE" effect known as death. Indeed, there are actually drugs that list death as a possible "side effect."

In other words, if a healthy person were to take ANY drug, they would be made ill.

Let us be very clear about one thing: *There are no such things as "side effects." These effects are direct and frontal assaults on your health.* Many times these side effects are worse than the original symptoms, and many symptoms known as "latter stages" of disease (cancer, "AIDS," diabetes, etc.) are in fact caused by these toxic and often lethal treatments.

DOES IT MAKE ANY SENSE TO GIVE A SICK PERSON A DRUG THAT WILL MAKE A HEALTHY PERSON SICK IN ORDER TO MAKE THE SICK PERSON HEALTHY.

It is very rare that a patient dies of cancer, despite what we are told. Most patients diagnosed with cancer die from the side effects of their highly toxic chemo-"therapy." Through the guise of "early detection saves lives," and fear-including admonitions by doctors and ignorant celebrities, more people than ever are being diagnosed and "treated" for cancer. Only in a very confused world would people subject themselves to having mustard gas injected in their veins, having breasts removed as a preventative measure, and succumbing to radiation "treatments" in hopes of becoming healthy, not to mention paying inordinate sums of money for these procedures. And the death rate from cancer (and cancer "treatments") continues to climb.

Our present and accepted methods of "healthcare" are

insane. In fact, *there is no such thing as true health care in modern medicine;* there is only disease classification, disease management and drug salesmanship. Doctors, in their concentration on disease, are blind to the ways of health, and hospitals lack EVERY essential for our well-being. Without sunshine or fresh air, hospitals offer toxic, disease-producing foods and drinks, daily druggings, and "treatments" and an atmosphere of patient powerlessness. A "good" (meaning obedient) patient has a much less chance to get out alive or unscathed as the patient with mind of his or her own.

DOCTORS ARE UNSCHOOLED IN HEALTH

I am first in line to applaud and admire the medical techniques, procedures, and skills of the doctors that mend broken bones, damaged tendons, and torn cartilage. Their skills and artistry in this area of reconstruction and structural repair are a tremendous boon to our civilization, allowing people to live their lives with greater comfort and ability. However, as far as their perspective on and treatment of disease goes, there is little to admire.

Doctors study disease (health failure) and drug use. Because of the constant influx of new drugs to replace the old ones that do not work, their education depends on the drug salesmen who represent the very companies that profit from the doctor's prescriptions. It is common practice for salesmen to give away free samples and offer perks such as free vacations, clock radios, and other gifts to doctors if they can sell a certain amount of new product. Drug companies will pay in full for luxurious vacations at the finest resorts and will invite scores of doctors and hospital administrators in order to "educate" them on the benefits of their new products.

The following is a list of direct quotes from a man who practiced medicine for more than thirty years. He is no longer with us, but his words are as valuable as ever to those who are committed to regaining their health and protecting their families and loved ones.

> *Whenever you are in hospital, you are in mortal danger.*
> *One of the unwritten rules of modern medicine is always to write a prescription for new drugs quickly before all its side effects have come to the surface.*
> *Doctors are not trained to attack the core of any problem, merely to suppress the symptoms.*
> *Doctors should be treated with about the same amount of trust as a used car salesman.*
> *I believe that more than ninety percent of modern medicine could disappear from the face of the earth—doctors, hospitals, drugs, and equipment—and the effect on our health would be immediate and beneficial.*
>
> —Dr. Robert Mendelsohn,
> *Confessions of a Medical Heretic*

Dr. Mendelsohn was an associate professor at the University of Illinois Medical School and the director of Chicago's Michael Reese Hospital. He wrote a syndicated column called *The People's Doctor* and was chairman of the Medical Licensure Committee for the state of Illinois. This man was educated by and worked in heart of the medical establishment. His efforts to report what other doctors deny and keep secret are a testament to his courage and veracity. He was a heroic man with a sense of decency who truly honored his physician's creed: FIRST, DO NO HARM. There are so few doctors who are willing to tell the truth about their profession (and apparently so few patients that ever question them) because the doctors who do inevitably suffer persecution and vilification from the AMA and mainstream society. These are some of the doctors who have stood up for truth and the healing powers of Nature's laws, despite the grave consequences and denigration they undoubtedly endured:

- Dr. John Tilden

- Dr. Russell Trall
- Dr. Sylvester Graham
- Dr. Issac Jennings
- Dr. Susanna W. Dodds
- Dr. William Alcott
- Dr. Joel Shew
- Dr. T.V. Gifford
- Dr. James Caleb Jackson
- Dr. Robert Willner

Doctors pour drugs of which they know little—to cure diseases of which they know less—into human beings of which they know nothing.

—Voltaire

There are a few doctors who presently are willing to be truthful about all they do not know and the dangerous practices of modern medicine, and they are vigorously persecuted for their honesty.

Our mechanical reaction to seek out a doctor for health advice needs to be fully examined if we are serious about our well-being.

Let us say you wanted to learn how to sing. Would you seek out an auto mechanic to teach you? Of course not. That is an absurd idea, as auto mechanics (as a rule) are not schooled in the art of voice and would be unable to help you attain the necessary skills. You would seek out somebody who is an expert vocalist. **If health is what you want, why would you go to somebody who studies the failure of heath (disease)?** If you wanted to become a millionaire would you go to skid row to interview the homeless and destitute about their financial planning skills?

If you were interested in health, it would make sense to STUDY HEALTH. The problem is that our perception of what health actually is remains quite distorted, and the possibility exists that we really do not have a human model for health. Certainly, modern medicine's use of a "normal" man or woman (feeding on unnatural foods and poisoning themselves forty to fifty times a day) as a model for health is baseless and absurd.

The intention of this work is to provide the reader with a sane and logical guideline to health. The problems that exist concerning health are listed as well as the solutions.

The program is simple yet quite challenging to those of the civilized, fast food, quick-fix world, but it is *unimaginably* rewarding. It is also cheap, convenient, and wonderfully effective—see for yourself.

There is also no pressure to do this immediately or completely. You might want to make some diligent efforts to incorporate some of these principles and see for yourself if your health and vitality does not improve.

I remember the days when I first came across this knowledge of natural feeding and thought how sensible and logical it sounded, despite the fact that I was eating close to the Standard American Diet (or SAD). I thought how difficult it was going to be to give up my favorite foods, i.e., pizza, cheeseburgers, ice cream, etc.

> *There are more things in heaven and earth than are dreamt of in your philosophies.*
>
> —Shakespeare

Yes, I can honestly tell you that the very foods I dreaded giving up are presently completely unappealing to me, and many of them seem downright disgusting. I am in disbelief about many of the things I used to eat on a daily basis. Certainly, if somebody told me twenty years ago that I would be a raw foodist and no longer eat the foods I was so completely attached to and be completely content, I would have told them that they were nuts. I had no reference at the time for this way of living and all its life-enhancing, exquisite benefits. You may be in the same situation. Give this program a try; you can always go back to your former ways.

There was a friend of mine who would periodically talk to me about the harmful effects of animal products, and I responded with impatience, disrespect, and often-lighthearted ridicule about the one or two vegetarians I knew. This was my short-sighted, uninformed impression of the knowledge that was being offered to me, and I wanted no part of it. **As my willingness to hear the truth increased, so did my health and happiness.**

It is very difficult for us to hear information that challenges our comfort zones and settled ideas. However, making these kinds of efforts is SO essential to our overall growth as human beings, and so tremendously exciting with results that are almost immediately measurable. It is a wonderful thing to UNDERSTAND health and live according to the Laws of Nature; to eat with consciousness and no longer add to the suffering that is so rampant on our planet, to no longer partake of foods that are destroying our ecology and our health, and to no longer feel at the mercy of disease or fear old age and the onset of a debilitated body. What a gift it would be to find a lifestyle that provides one with near autonomy over one's health.

If you or a loved one have been told that you are doomed to live with an "incurable" or "chronic" disease, you have been lied to. You do not have to suffer through the drugging, burnings, poisonings, mutilations, irradiations, and hopelessness prescribed to you. You now have the opportunity to do what thousands of others have done; you can take responsibility for your wellbeing and understand the true nature of disease and the simplicity of health and allow your body to do what it knows best—heal.

Health is our natural state. Nothing needs to be added to gain health. It makes no sense to attempt to "gain" health by any kind of an addition to an already perfect mechanism. The steps that need to be taken to return to our intended state of health involve subtraction of harmful practices that create disease. The following two chapters on meat and dairy products, two of our most widely used and damaging food products, suggest great places to start subtracting.

Chapter 1

----- ❖ ◆ ❖ -----

THE DISASTER OF ANIMAL PRODUCTS

It is my view that the vegetarian manner of living, by its purely physical effect on the human temperament, would most beneficial influence the lot of mankind.

—Albert Einstein

For the first twenty years of my life I was raised on the Standard American Diet (SAD), and I rarely, if ever, questioned the idea of what I was ingesting. I loved bacon, cheeseburgers, ham, steak, and all the "normal" foods that our society accepts. I also believed these foods were necessary for my health and well-being. It is a common belief that eating animal products is essential for building muscle and keeping our strength up. As an athlete, I certainly did not want to jeopardize my strength or ability to build muscle, and I did not begin to seriously question what I ate until the age of twenty-one.

Being a meat-eater for such a long period of time makes it difficult to judge anybody for the unconscious eating habits that I, myself, practiced for years. This information had not found me yet, and, in my ignorance, there was no problem with the way I was living my life, blind to the truth of what eating animals entailed and all its catastrophic consequences. I was completely trusting of what I had been told; I did as others did. Having knowledge of the information that follows made it impossible for me to continue on, thankfully so. Leaving off the eating of animals has deepened my compassion for ALL life on Earth and has made a huge impact on the quality of my health.

Certainly the following chapter may be disturbing; there is no doubt that many people do not want to read about the accepted mayhem and brutality that our society condones and supports. Indeed, it was not very popular to be one of the first abolitionists, back when slavery was accepted and unquestioned by the masses. According to many, even "men of God," certain colored men were supposed to own different colored men. If you were a woman and wanted to vote one hundred years ago, most people would think that you were a "radical" or a "revolutionist," as the idea of a woman voting was offensive. These were the time-honored, conventional practices of the day and were not to be questioned.

Is there any doubt that those who were brave enough to originally express their opposition to these perverse practices were scoffed at and ridiculed for their conscientious opposition? Will there come a time when the present day heinous disregard and brutal treatment of animals are viewed with the same indignation and disgust we have today toward slavery and discrimination?

The following pages, which focus on the treacherous effects of our animal-based diet, are written with the intention of shining light on all that has been in the dark and hidden from mainstream society for so many years. It is shocking information.

Shocks are often necessary to awaken a sleeping public.

The films our country saw on the Vietnam War completely changed the way we view war. Because of the daily documentation of the atrocities of this particular war, the reality of war itself was made real in the minds of our citizens. It was no longer some type innocuous John Wayne movie where the good guys beat the bad guys. The pictures told the real and graphic story of the hell that war is. Because of this shock, public outcry against the war increased, and the war was mercifully ended years before it might have been without that revealing media exposure.

There is an equally atrocious, vile, and violent set of circumstances that exist today, the scope of which has yet to be realized by the general population. For whatever reasons these events have gone unnoticed and have remained hidden from the mainstream. We are all doing the best we can with what we know, and I believe that our existence here on Earth would change dramatically if we were more informed.

Please read the following with an open and objective mind and see if it makes sense to you. It may be uncomfortable to read against your intellectual and emotional attachments, but remember that all improvements (of yourself and the world) require significant and consistent effort and a certain degree of discomfort. These noble efforts that go against our comfort zones and heighten our consciousness are the very struggles that advance us as individuals and as people and, as such, are the only genuinely lasting rewards of life on Earth.

PROTEIN

"Where do you get your protein?" This is the most commonly posed question to those who leave off the eating of animals and eat according to the Laws of Nature. It is best answered with a series of other questions: Where does a horse get its protein? Where does an ox get its protein? Where does a rhinoceros or an elephant get its protein? **All of these incredibly muscular and powerful animals are herbivores that eat nothing but plant life, yet they have immense strength and vitality.**

It is true that these animals have a physiology that is quite different from that of a human being. However, THE strongest mammal on the planet is the silverback gorilla, who has an almost identical digestive system to ours, and the many physiological similarities between our two species are quite evident. Despite being anywhere from two to three times as large as a human being, these gorillas are thirty times as strong. These animals have an incredibly powerful physique and ingest nothing but plant life.

How is it and why is it that our society is so convinced that we need to ingest a large amount of protein and animal products to be strong and healthy while the example nature sets goes unnoticed? We eat the flesh of a cow for protein, yet all the cow eats in its natural environment is the grass. If all aforementioned animals feed themselves exclusively with plant life, why is it that we are so concerned with "getting enough protein?"

HAVE YOU EVER HEARD OF ANYBODY WITH A PROTEIN DEFICIENCY?

The protein myth has been developed, like all myths, by people repeating things they been told instead of verifying those ideas as factual for themselves.

This is an old and reliable recipe for brainwashing the masses. "Realities" are formed by collective agreement and often have nothing to do with the truth.

We do not have to think too far back to remember the days of the oft-mentioned "four food groups," two of which were "meat and dairy" products. One would be hard pressed to find one of these pamphlets or food charts that was not put together by the

REPEAT A LIE LONG ENOUGH AND LOUD ENOUGH AND IT BECOMES A REALITY.

meat industry or the dairy council. As far as the "reality" of the four food groups goes, there is absolutely NO scientific, physiological or biological evidence to support this recommended nutritional guideline that our doctors and physicians embarrassingly promulgated for more than thirty years. This salesmanship by certain businesses and backed by "health professionals" has caused untold numbers of diseased, dying, and dead citizens.

Mercifully, the "four food groups" fiasco has ended; yet the myth of getting enough protein continues to grow and hover in the unconscious belief system of the masses. It is a wonderful marketing ploy to scare the unknowing public into believing that they need to have a certain food product or their health will deteriorate. It is especially effective when "experts" repeat the lies in order to sell specious products, much the same way doctors used to recommend and advertise cigarettes to the television audiences of the fifties and sixties, obviously helping to increase the possibility of lung cancer and death in exchange for a few bucks from the tobacco companies.

Scientifically speaking, the definition of a protein is a chain link of amino acids. In other words: **amino acids are the building blocks of protein.**

According to our scientists there are twenty-three different types of amino acids, eight of which they claim are "essential." They are ALL essential. According to our present scientists, the body produces fifteen amino acids, and the other eight must be derived from our food intake. If you are eating even a small array of fruits, you are receiving every amino acid and nutrient you need, just as animals in nature are well nourished as they abide by their instincts.

There is no greater source, in terms of both quantity and quality, for amino acids than raw fruits and vegetables and raw seeds and nuts. These are the same fruits and vegetables our plant-eating animal friends in their natural environment use to build their amazing bodies and strength. There are no supplements or protein powders. No animals weigh their food or add up their protein/ carbohydrate intake and no animals eat according to their blood type. Are the power, vitality, and health of these species proof enough that nature has provided all the nutrients we need with plant food? Perhaps this evidence is logical and sensible to those who can TRULY think for themselves, an almost impossible task in our well-programmed society.

The most perfect human food on the planet, mother's milk, has only three percent protein. This food, designed by the Supreme Creator, is the food infants can eat exclusively to grow their bodies in the first years of life on Earth. It is a complete and perfect food, providing the mother is in good health, and is a clear indication that protein is not the most important nutrient for a human being.

Flesh foods provide no fuel or energy. In fact, despite the often stimulating effects of meat, it is incredibly devitalizing and enervating to the human body. It takes tremendous energy to digest flesh foods, and one of the natural by-products of cooked animal flesh digestion is ammonia. The amino are acids that carnivorous animals use to build their bodies (while eating the raw meat, of course) are coagulated and destroyed through the process of cooking. Not only is meat a poor source of protein, it is toxic to the body and is disease-producing. Even the AMA has documented the cancer causing effects of ingesting cooked animal flesh. The Journal of the National Cancer Institute says, "'Heart disease' deaths and bowel cancer deaths are directly proportional to meat consumption." The National Cancer Research Institute found that women who eat daily portions of meat are four times more likely to get breast cancer than those women who eat little or no meat.

Animal products are the prime source of the cholesterol that clogs arteries. If it were recognized, this is a fact that could immediately cut in half the number of those suffering from heart disease. Of course, **the elimination of polyunsaturated fat and hydrogenated oils found in margarine and other "low fat" highly processed foods, along with the cessation of ingesting animal products, would end the epidemic of arteriosclerosis, stroke, and heart attacks from which we suffer.**

Evidence of the benefits of a vegetarian diet has been well documented. The healthiest people in the world, the Hunzukuts, (or Hunzas) commonly live past the age of one hundred, stay extremely active their entire lives, and rarely experience any disease. There are no formula drinks, no steroids, and no osteoporosis. These people have been examined by western doctors such as Dr. Alexander Leaf, who did a study for National Geographic on the oldest people in the world and the illustrious and prominent physician Dr. Paul Dudley White, who tended to President Eisenhower. Besides finding no obesity, no cancer and no diabetes, they found no heart disease. Dr. White did a study on twenty-five men over the age of ninety and found them to be in perfect health. The Hunzas diet is strictly vegetarian and consists of eighty percent raw food.

The Pythagoreans, Buddhists, Taoists, and the Essenes all regarded a vegetarian diet as a necessary discipline. In fact, according to many Biblical scholars such as Ernest Renan (*Life of Jesus*), Jesus Christ himself was an Essene and a vegetarian. From the Essene Gospel of Peace, Christ is quoted, "Eat nothing to which the fire of death gives savor, for such is Satan."

Many people will say, "Human beings have been eating meat for thousands of years." Maybe that is true, maybe not, as some anthropologists claim that the first human beings were exclusively fruit eaters. The argument could be made that we have also been murdering and torturing each other as well as waging wars for thousands of years, right up to and through the present day "civilized" world. These are practices that need to be examined. Just because we have been doing something for a long time does not mean it should not be questioned.

Let us take an objective look at this practice of killing and eating animals.

Physiologically speaking, there are clear and inarguable differences between the physical makeup of a carnivore and a human being. The first is the obvious lack of foot speed we have compared to flesh-eating animals. Every flesh eater is equipped with great speed and/or blinding quickness. The fastest human being in the world is nowhere near as fast as wild cats or dogs.

All carnivores' jaws are extremely powerful and move exclusively up and down which is extremely effective for ripping and tearing flesh. Plant eaters have jaws that move not only up and down but also from side to side. This functional difference is plain to see in the animal kingdom.

Carnivores have fangs and claws effectively designed to inflict fatal wounds on their prey. We do not. Could you imagine trying to kill an animal without a gun, a knife, or some other type of weapon? Many carnivores have the strength and ability to bring down animals that are two to three times their size and weight. Their ability to kill is built in; they need nothing other than that with which they were born. We cannot say that about our own physiology. Imagine yourself confronting a full-sized deer, antelope, elephant, or giraffe with the intent to inflict a fatal blow. It would be a more-than-comical sight as well as quite dangerous to your well being. The animal might be somewhat confused at the sight of this harmless creature (you) standing before him, with bad intentions but obviously ill-equipped to murder, or even do any significant physical harm. Our physical strength is no match when compared to wild carnivorous animals.

There are those that claim that we have two canine teeth and argue that this is evidence that we were meant to eat meat. Let these people try to eat a raw piece of meat without the use of sharp knives, meat grinders, or food processors. Then we can discuss their findings. Our teeth and jaws are set up for the chewing mastication of plant life.

Our saliva is alkaline; carnivores have acidic saliva. Carnivores' stomachs secrete ten times the amount of hydrochloric acid than human beings do. Hydrochloric acid is the vital and necessary substance used for flesh digestion. Our digestive systems are completely different. Further, carnivores have rough abrasive tongues; ours are smooth.

Millions of Americans and citizens of other "civilized" countries suffer from the painful, debilitating condition known as rheumatism or arthritis. When an animal is slaughtered, all eliminative processes end at once, and the urine or uric acid that was marked for elimination remains in the flesh of the animal. Carnivores are equipped to deal with this ingested urine. They have an enzyme called uricase specifically designed for this purpose. Human beings do not have uricase. The massive amount of urine ingested by meat-eating humans is extremely difficult for our digestive system to process. After years of filthy, unnatural habit of ingesting the dead, the uric acid begins to crystallize in a human body and is deposited in the joints, causing the painful twisting and turning of the bones, stiffness, and lameness. Doctors claim this condition to be "incurable." I have seen this condition repeatedly reversed and eliminated by those who end their carnivorous habits.

The intestines of a carnivorous animal are extremely short, only about three times the length of its body, so that the unused ingested flesh food is dispelled quickly and the decaying flesh does not linger in the digestive tract of the animal. Human beings have intestines that reach twelve times the length of their trunk to allow for proper absorption of the needed nutrients derived from the ingested plant life. Flesh food in our digestive tract is a disaster, incredibly difficult and sometimes impossible to digest. Surgeons have reported that undigested flesh foods that do not break down will remain stuck or impacted in a patient's track for YEARS.

It is common for lions and tigers to sleep for twenty hours after feeding on flesh, an indication of the nerve energy used to break down their meal. It is also interesting to note that these carnivores do not eat other carnivores, and the first part of the vegetarian animal they eat is the intestines where all the water-rich plant life digests.

> *No human beings past the thoughtless age of boyhood will*
> *wantonly murder any creature which holds its life by the*
> *same tenure that he does.*
>
> —Thoreau

PSYCHOLOGICAL ASPECTS OF FLESH EATING

Please give some serious thought to the following questions:

- What is your first reaction upon seeing a dead animal?
- Are you interested?
- Do you have an impulse to get closer?
- Do you want to smell the stinking carcass?
- Do you want to taste it?
- Have you ever drooled at the sight of road kill?
- Does the sight of a dead animal increase, or decrease your appetite?
- Isn't your first reaction to bloodied, dead animal revulsion?

The answers to these questions are obvious. Human beings are disgusted and repelled by the sight of dead, bloodied animals. As soon as the life force is ended, a body immediately begins to decompose and rot, causing a foul stench and an ugly sight which is not very appetizing. Sure enough, this sight creates disgust in us and a natural instinct to stay away. This is hard to deny. Strangely enough these rotting, decaying cadavers have become the main "food" in our civilized society's diet. WHY? How could this be if our natural instinct toward a rotting cadaver is utter disgust? The natural instinct of our cats and dogs IS to sniff it and inspect it; however, most wild cats and dogs will not eat a carcass unless it has just been killed. Somehow eating "aged" meat has become some kind of a delicacy for our "civilized society." Only nature's scavengers, including vultures, hyenas, flies, etc., will indulge in a rotting corpse. **Human beings are not meant to be scavengers,** and it is a blow to our dignity to partake in this filthy food and act as scavengers. "Don't touch it!" is what we yell to our children when coming across an animal corpse; we then walk to the picnic table and give them a corpse sandwich to eat.

Perhaps it is a bit unnerving or even shocking to refer to a hamburger or turkey sandwich as a "corpse" sandwich; yet that is exactly what it is. An apple is an apple, an orange is an orange, and a rotting decaying piece of flesh is a corpse. Eating a corpse is a ghoulish act. Of course we are not inclined to think in this manner and have invented many wonderful euphemisms for these animal cadavers. These linguistic niceties provide us with buffers and distract us from paying attention to just what it is that we eat on a daily basis. We do not eat sliced cadavers; we eat cold cuts, hot dogs or hamburgers.

Confucius once said, when being asked how to uplift a fallen society, that the first order of business is to "rectify the language." This wise man understood that language could be used to control the populace and make them do things that are disastrous to their well being. Language plays a huge role in the hypnotizing the masses. For instance, in this country we have a "Defense" Department that wages war. It used to be called the War department. The "Defense" Department now refers to the battlefield as the "theater," kills as "casualties," and wars as "conflicts." **We have a "healthcare" system in charge of disease management that knows nothing about health** and "side effects" that can kill. George Orwell, in his novel *1984*, predicted that by the end of the twentieth century language would be used as such a successful weapon against the people ("newspeak") that free speech and freedom of choice would not be possible.

The people who sell dead animals for food, along with our entire society, have agreed to an ingenious and impressive array of euphemisms to deal with the common practice of feeding on the dead. There are few people who would return to a restaurant if a steak were listed on the menu as "Dead Cow" or "Rotting Cadaver." That would not be polite. When selling treacherous products it is not good business to be candid or direct.

We are in the habit of invoking the romantic languages of France and Italy and other countries to eat and sell cadavers as food: "filet mignon," "chateaubriand," "foie gras," (fat liver), "veal scaloppini," "filet of sole," "steak tartare," "escargot" (snails). Most people would not eat snails on a dare, let alone pay thirty or forty bucks for this "delicacy," unless it is carried with it the pretentious air of "sophistication" that it does. Next time you are in a restaurant, it might be interesting to order your food using plain language: "I'll have the dead baby cow and the liver of a tortured goose with a glass of spoiled (fermented) red grape juice." Your waiter might give you a strange look, your friends could be disgusted, and you also might end up ordering a salad. Everyone will profit.

> *You have just dined; and however scrupulously the slaughterhouse is concealed in the graceful distance of miles, there is complicity.*
>
> —Emerson

I wonder how many people would be able to go out hack

to death a docile, peaceful cow, sift through the gallons of blood and guts, and tear away some flesh to put upon the stove every time they wanted a hamburger, a roast beef sandwich, a hot dog, or a steak.

What if our children understood that hamburgers do not "grow in patches" as McDonalds would have them believe? What if they knew the fright and sheer terror these animals experienced before their execution? What if they knew the rush of adrenalin and fear that courses through the blood of these beings before they are slaughtered, and that the hamburgers they eat are filled with that adrenaline and fear?

IF WE WERE OBLIGED TO KILL EVERY TIME WE WANTED A PIECE OF MEAT, HOW WOULD THAT AFFECT THE DIETARY HABITS OF OUR CULTURE?

What if they knew that these animals were tortured their entire lives and suffered a horrific execution, being hung upside down by one leg, which immediately dislocates and often breaks, at which point their throats are cut until they slowly bleed to death. Perhaps they would understand that becoming an Oscar Meyer wiener (as the song goes) is not what they would wish for after all. Maybe they would not want to order their "Happy Meals" with such frequency. Maybe they would see that they are in fact Horror Meals and be rightfully afraid and unwilling to partake in such fiercely inhumane and brutally slaughtered gore.

> The time will come when men such as I will look on the murder of animals as they now look on the murder of men.
>
> —Leonardo da Vinci

The fact is that not just our children but our entire population is carefully and intentionally kept very far from the harsh, nightmarish brutality that goes on every day in this country. **There are ten million animals a day put to death in this country alone.** Despite that staggering number of killings, not many of us have ever seen what goes on inside a slaughterhouse. Why is it that we are so far removed from these places of death if flesh eating is such a major and completely accepted part of our lives? The answer is simple: It would be too horrible a sight for most of our population to bear.

Animals can hear the screams, smell the stench, and often see the cows being put to death before them. Dr. Temple Grandin reports numerous cases of "deliberate cruelty" from the workers who "enjoy killing and tormenting animals on purpose," taking "sadistic pleasure from shooting the eyes out of cattle, striking them in the head, and electrically shocking them in sensitive areas of their bodies." Before their throats are cut these animals are hit with a pistol bolt set against the side of their head, and a metal rod is mechanically shot into the brain. Because the animal is often upset and fighting for its life, the bolt misses its mark, creating tremendous pain.

> *I saw with my own eyes innocent animals having their heads bashed in with a captive bolt pistol, some two or three times. Then a man would walk over and slit the cow's throat. Buckets of blood poured out. It was horrible – the animals were squirming and screaming. One of the men came out of a room while sharpening a knife and told us to watch out for cows that fall off the chain and charge the workers.*

—Mike Lace
Grant City, Illinois, April, 1997

> *A meat packing plant is like nothing you have ever seen or could imagine. It's like a vision of hell.*

—Eleanor Kennelly
United Food & Commercial Workers Union

It is uplifting to have seen so many people go out of their

way to take in abused and abandoned animals and compassionately spend their time and money finding loving homes for these unfortunate dogs and cats. However, it is an incongruous bizarre event to see these very people eat a hot dog or hamburger without a thought of the life of violence and abuse a cow or pig endures.

It is astonishing how many people love their pets as if they were family members, appreciating their personalities, extending their kindness, and sustaining loving relationships with them. They protect them from harm and go to great lengths to treat them when they are sick or injured; but then these people turn around and support and partake in the brutalization of other species by buying and eating animal products. If these people were to treat their house-pets the way farm animals are treated, they would immediately be arrested and shunned by the public for their heartless cruelty.

Many people are addicted to the "taste" of flesh foods, unaware that the taste they are actually enjoying is the steak sauces and seasonings used in the preparation. These days there are many vegetarian "meat substitutes" available to those who crave this certain texture and taste, and if you use the same dressings and preparations, you will not be able to tell the difference. A shiitake mushroom grilled and sauced up will satisfy most meat eaters. Veggie burgers taste much better than any flesh burger; indeed, it is hard to tell the difference between the two, and just think, there's no blood in your burger!

The greatness of a nation and its moral progress can be judged by the way its animals are treated.

—Gandhi

If the great physiological and psychological damage we perpetrate by eating flesh are not reason enough for us to consider ending this malefic practice, maybe the following will provide some added incentive.

Before you order veal scaloppini again, here is something you might want to know. In order to bring that white flesh to your plate, a very sadistic operation takes place on a farm. The calf is pulled from its mother after birth. Cows are driven mad by the abduction of their child and have been known to kick holes in cement walls. The calf is chained and shackled to a tiny stall where the animal is unable to move, turn around, or lie down comfortably. Frightened and alone, desperate to suckle on anything and feel the connection with its mother, this calf is forced to live in its own filth and excrement, forced to spend its entire existence in the dark, forced-fed an artificial drug-laced diet, and intentionally driven to anemia before it is slaughtered. Most of the industrialized farms, which make up the majority of farms house cattle in row houses the length of football fields, in which the animals never see the light of day or touch their hoofs to the earth. They are kept on a steel grate their entire existence, which causes painful deformities and injuries to their hoofs and legs. They are fed and injected with drugs, steroids and antibiotics, and constantly sprayed with toxic pesticides in the course of their agonizing lives. The commonly sprayed pesticide toxaphene, according to the US Environmental Protection Agency, is so toxic that a few parts per billion will dissolve the bones of an animal. This deadly poison is absorbed into the flesh of these animals.

There are NO doctors or pharmaceutical experts that can predict, in terms of the danger or "side effects," what happens when you mix two drugs together, let alone the ten to twenty pharmaceuticals with which these cows are often fed and injected. These cattle are being pumped with drugs for their entire lives. However, scientists do know that something called THMs (trihalomethanes) are formed when mixing drugs. THMs are a known carcinogen.

The three thousand doctors that make up the Physicians Committee for Responsible Medicine estimate the annual health care costs resulting directly from meat consumption to be somewhere between $23.6 billion and $61.4 billion.

Penicillin is commonly fed to and injected into farm animals. Many human beings can die from an allergic reaction to this commonly used, highly toxic drug. How much more penicillin does the cow need compared to a human being? Obviously a considerable amount more, considering that cows are eight to ten times our size. Because of the unnatural, bizarre environment these cattle (also chickens and pigs) are raised in, the frequency of the drugging is quite high. So there are extremely high doses of a drug that can kill human beings in much smaller doses, frequently administered to millions of farm animals that we commonly eat. There are no warnings to the public, no labels listing the plethora of drugs that come with each pound of ground beef, chicken leg, slice of bacon or hotdog, and there is hardly any objection from the public.

Steroids and growth hormones, sadly enough, are being used by many of today's professional and amateur athletes. These strength and performance enhancers are directly related to resulting aggressive, antisocial and violent behavior. Anabolic steroids are implanted in the ears of cattle in the form of time-release pellets. These hormones seep into the blood stream and increase hormone levels by two to five times. According to an article in the *National Food Review* (July–Sep, 1989), more than ninety-five percent of feedlot-raised cattle in the US are currently being administered growth promoting hormones.

Could the conclusion be made that most of our citizens are ingesting steroids on a daily basis? How does this affect the way we treat one another? Could the violence in our society have anything to do with the ingesting of steroids? I have been around many athletes on steroids; the mood swings and aggressive behavior are quite evident. Trial attorneys have been known to use the defense, "My client was on steroids at the time of the crime."

I doubt even the heartiest meat eater on the planet would not be affected by the following. The FDA and USDA allow and approve the following to be used as feed for farm animals: chicken feces, cow feces, ground-up cardboard, cement dust, ammonia, "plastic hay," body parts of chickens and cows and IRRADIATED SEWAGE SLUDGE. They actually take sewage sludge and expose it to nuclear fallout (CZM 176, cobalt 60) and use it as feed.

The results—many people eat this poisoned flesh and die immediately, or a few days after ingestion. Our medical experts have the nerve to blame these deaths, violent seizures, and sickness that meat eaters increasingly experience on salmonella or e–coli bacteria, never mentioning the concentration of toxins, deadly pharmaceuticals, pesticides, steroids and growth hormones, or irradiated sewage sludge found in these animal products.

WOULD PEOPLE KNOWINGLY INGEST AND PAY FOR SUCH A SICKENING ARRAY OF INGREDIENTS, OR IS DECEPTION AND MISREPRESEN- TAION NECESSARY FOR PROFIT?

These sentient beings are treated with no dignity or compassion and live an agonizing, unnatural existence filled with disease and physical pain. It is no wonder that few, if any, of our citizens are ever exposed to the brutal and cruel existence these animals endure. I wonder how many people would change their diet if they spent five minutes on the kill floor of a slaughterhouse amongst the screaming animals, chopped-off heads, and rivers of blood.

Life on the farm is no better for chickens. They are commonly kept in two-by-two-foot cages, six to a cage. They have their beaks sawed off (an agonizing event), are driven insane by this torturous existence, often resorting to pecking each other's eyes out and killing one another. They are unable to move; their nails grow around the cages, and they are fed a steady diet of antibiotics and pharmaceuticals along with poisoned and toxic feeds.

Our leaders speak about the violence on TV and in movies as being a main cause of the violence in our society. This violence on the screen is portrayed by actors playing roles and saying lines from a script. It may seem very real and may in fact desensitize a viewer to violent acts. However, these actors all go home intact and unharmed; it is pretend violence. Does it have an impact? There is a possibility that it does, and according to some hard evidence, pretend violence does affect the way we treat each other. But the unseen, unrealizable murder and mayhem that goes on EVERY DAY in these slaughterhouses is REAL VIOLENCE that makes a Freddy Krueger movie look like *Sesame Street.*

> *Non-violence leads to the highest ethics, which is the goal of all evolution. Until we stop harming all other living beings, we are all still savages.*
>
> —Thomas Edison

Many Americans are shocked at the heinous treatment of dogs in Korea and other dog-eating countries. These dogs exist in the most deplorable and inhumane conditions and are often intentionally terrified before they are slaughtered to "make the meat taste better." Our population thinks it reprehensible and outrageously cruel to treat man's best friend with such indignity and cruelty, and those "dog-eaters" are viewed as barbaric and wicked human beings by our civilized society. Apparently, our civilized culture has the inside information on what are the proper animals—cows, pigs, fish, and chickens—to torture and slaughter and has no hesitation supporting the millions of daily murders.

Can any human being really appreciate what ten million daily killings entail? Do we have the capacity to feel for and understand the amount of pain and agony that is inflicted on these animals daily? Just because they are animals we have not met, does it mean that it is all right to abuse and slaughter them? Does this have an effect on how we view the suffering of other human beings? Can we calculate the effects of this daily sadistic inhumanity and the impact it has on our population? No, it is quite obvious that we would be overwhelmed in our attempts to really appreciate all these issues, all the beings, and all the agonies endured. It is not possible for us.

Remember that this is REAL violence, not violence acted out on a screen for our viewing pleasure. Real violence that takes place millions of times each day. Real violence has real consequences. The vibratory thrust of this daily holocaust hangs heavily over our populace and has grave repercussions for us all. Would anyone doubt that the cessation of torturing and killing animals would have a tremendously uplifting effect on our culture?

Niccolo Machiavelli, the Renaissance diplomat and tactician, when commenting on pagan people and their rituals reported the following:

> Their ceremonies lacked neither pomp nor magnificence, but they added the extremely bloody and fierce act of sacrifice in which hordes of animals were killed. This savage aspect of them tended to make the participants savage too.

Remember that every time you buy a product you are voting. What does it say about society that we, in an overwhelming majority vote for and support this daily animal abuse? Do you want to continue voting this way because it "tastes good?"

You might want to ask yourself, "Is it really the taste of the meat I enjoy, or is it the texture, salt, pepper, spices, herbs, and other flavorings that I enjoy?" "Is it the emotional ties and familiarity to which I've grown so accustomed?" "Would I be doing myself and the rest of the world, including my family, a big favor by finding other comfort foods?"

If you have any doubt whether you can be as strong and as powerful as you like on a vegetarian diet, and the examples of the Herculean strength of nature's animals (rhinoceros, ox, horse, elephant, gorilla, etc.) are not enough, here is a list of great human athletes that left off the eating of animals:

Carl Lewis: Maybe the greatest athlete ever, won a total of nine Olympic gold medals and numerous world championships. He held world records in 100-meter dash and 400-meter relay. The one-time "fastest man in the world" would consistently beat a field of drug-enhanced challengers. He may be the last pure track star of our time.

Edwin Moses: World and Olympic champion who went eight years without losing a race in the 400-meter hurdles. He is possibly the most dominant athlete of his time. *Sports Illustrated* Athlete of the Year 1984.

Bill Walton: Basketball player. He may be the most dominant collegiate center ever, winning four NCAA championships at UCLA. Walton went on to win NBA championships with the Portland Trail Blazers and the Boston Celtics.

Murray Rose: Three-time gold medalist in the 1956 Olympics. Four years later came back to become the first man to retain his 400-meter freestyle title; he broke his own world record in the 400- and 1500-meter freestyle. Rose has been a vegetarian since he was two years old.

Lou Savarese: Professional prizefighter. He has been ranked in top ten heavyweights in the world.

Andreas Cahling: Swedish body builder who won the Mr. International title in 1980 and competed for 10 years at the highest level of body building competition.

Dave Scott: Won the Ironman Triathlon four times.

Roy Hilligan: A vegetarian bodybuilder who won the Mr. America title.

Stan Price: A power lifter who held the world record for bench press in his weight class.

Bill Pearl: World-famous body builder and lifting guru.

According to Grecian lore, Milos of Croton, a Pythagorean disciple, was a legendary wrestler who never lost a match. He was a victor in five successive Olympiads in the sixth century B.C., and the story goes that he was never brought to his knees.

This list can go on a lot longer, but the point is well made. Whether it is pure strength, physical toughness, endurance, skill, speed, or a combination of them all, this list of great athletes is evidence enough that vegetarians lose nothing by leaving off the eating of animals.

I am convinced that as soon as one major athlete recognized the benefits of not just vegetarianism or veganism, but raw foodism and begins to abide by the Laws of Nature, other athletes will quickly follow.

FISH

There are many people who call themselves vegetarians and continue to eat fish. I have yet to see a plant grow a fish. I have often heard people who come across an unpleasant odor exclaim with disgust and offensive distaste, "It smells like fish in here." I do not know too many people who find the look or smell of fish, let alone the scaly texture, appealing or inviting, not to mention appetizing. Walking by a fishery on the pier can be a sickening experience if you do not have some heavy cloth to press against your nose to protect you from the gag-inducing, putrid stench. If someone were to plunk a dead fish into your lap right now, what would your initial, instinctive reaction be?

In spite of our natural aversion to the presence of dead fish, we are happy to order our well-cooked and carefully prepared "filet of sole." It really is quite an amazing trick we play on ourselves, and it makes me wonder if there is **no limit** to what we might eat if it were presented in the right way. This stinking fish we want to get away from as fast as possible somehow becomes an item we want on our dinner plate, and we gladly pay for it. Conversely, if someone threw an apple on your lap, you might thank them.

The Center for Disease Control claims an average of 325,000 reports of food poisoning from fish each year. If that is what is reported, one has to wonder how many more poisonings go unreported. Due to our heavily polluted oceans, lakes, and rivers, most fish contain mercury, an extremely toxic metal substance that can destroy the nervous system and cause grave illness. There are only a few areas where fish are not living in mercury-tainted waters.

In addition to mercury, it is more than common that the fish on our plates have large amounts of PCBs. A synthetic liquid used for industrial purposes, this baneful carcinogen was outlawed in 1976. A six-month investigation done by Consumers Union revealed that, "By far the biggest source of PCBs in the human diet is fish," and "The PCBs you eat today will be with you for decades into the future." Ingesting PCBs causes reduced sperm counts in men and may be related to birth defects.

Many environmental experts and oceanographers have given stern warnings to humanity about the over-fishing that is destroying the homeostasis of our oceans. High-tech industrial fishing methods, including sonar and spotting planes, have enabled commercial fishers to vacuum up eighty to ninety percent of the entire fish populations in one year's time. The United Nations has reported that all seventeen major fishing areas on our planet have either reached or exceeded their natural limits. Just as we are clear-cutting and annihilating our rainforests, we are razing and pillaging our oceans. Two of our most precious resources are being devastated because we insist on an animal-based diet. A shocking fact (from *Scientific American*, Nov. 1995) and another reason to stop eating animals is that **one-third of all caught fish are turned into fish-meal** for livestock.

If our oceans make up seventy percent of our planet and they and are being destroyed and polluted, how does that impact the rest of our environment?

LAND USAGE AND STARVING CHILDREN

Besides wreaking havoc on our bodies and compromising our conscience, our animal-based diet is a main factor in the destruction of our planet and also one of the main contributing factors in the hunger and starvation of millions.

From a recent *Sierra Club* article (1999):

> *A December 1997 report prepared for Iowa Senator Tom Harkin (D), who sits on the Senate Committee on Agriculture, says that animal waste is the largest contributor to pollution in 60 percent of the rivers and streams classified as "impaired" by the Environmental Protection Agency. According to the same report, the United States generates 1.4 billion tons of animal manure every year—130 times more than the annual production of human waste. Cattle manure leads the list at 1.2 billion tons, followed by pig manure at 116 million tons, and chicken manure at 14 million tons.*

One third of the world's total grain production goes to feed cattle. Less than half of the farm acreage in this country is now used to grow food for people. The livestock population of the U.S. consumes enough grains and soybeans to feed the American population five times over. The livestock population gets more than eighty percent of the corn and ninety-five percent of the oats we grow. One half of our water supply goes to cattle farming. Cattle outweigh human beings on the planet two to one. Yet we do not hear politicians or UN representatives address this growing population disaster, this locust-like swarm of cattle that is ravaging our planet; yet they continue to warn us of human overpopulation on a daily basis.

The more than one billion cattle on this planet produce more than one fifth of the environmental devastating methane gas responsible for the phenomenon known as global warming. At the turn of the nineteenth century, American farmland had topsoil that averaged twenty-one inches in depth. Today only six inches remain. That meat industry is responsible for more than eighty-five percent of the topsoil erosion in this country.

EVERY THREE SECONDS A CHILD DIES OF STARVATION.

In 1984, when thousands of people in Ethiopia were dying daily from starvation, that country continued to export grain and feed to European countries as cattle feed. There are currently millions of acres of Third World countries being exclusively used to produce feed for European cattle while many of their people starve to death. Malnutrition is the principle cause of death in many Third World countries. In many of these countries twenty-five percent of the population dies before the age of four. Guatemala exports forty million pounds of beef to the United States while seventy-five percent of their children under the age of five are undernourished. The conditions in Costa Rica and the rest of Central America are not much better.

This hunger and suffering that runs rampant throughout our world is not caused by any defect of nature. The pain, starvation, and death is caused by human beings who must be uninformed, disinterested, arrogant, greedy, or all of the above.

Yet we continue to prioritize the feeding of livestock. It is quite clear that, by living the way we presently do, and by making the food choices we presently make in our "civilized" countries, we are directly contributing to the savagery and brutality of mass starvation.

> *I tremble for my species when I reflect that God is just.*
>
> —Thomas Jefferson

The most precious lands on our planet are being systematically destroyed so we can have cheap hamburgers. Tropical rainforests across the globe are being annihilated to graze cattle, setting off a long, dangerous domino effect of ecological and environmental destruction. The current rate of species extinction is one thousand per year, and most of that is directly related to the destruction of these incredibly lush and vibrant rainforests that are an essential part of our planet's well being.

> *More than twenty-five percent of the forests in Central America have been cleared for pasture land, and most cattle produced is exported to developing countries for use in fast food hamburgers.*
>
> —Costa Rica Rainforest Outward Bound School, 1996

Mexico and Central America used to be covered by 160,000 square miles of tropical rainforests; they now are down to under 40,000 square miles as the clear cutting for cattle pastures continues. These forests have taken thousands of years to develop and are a major part of our eco-system. If this destruction continues, we may never recover.

Francis Moore Lappe, the author of the environmental classic *Diet for a Small Planet*, described how Caterpillar tractors are razing and annihilating the Latin America rainforests. "Gargantuan 35-ton D-9s mounted with angle plows weighing 2,500 pounds each bulldoze the forest at 2,700 yards an hour uprooting everything in sight." For every quarter pound hamburger that comes from a steer raised in Central and South America, it is necessary to destroy approximately 165 pounds of living matter.

In Plato's *Republic*, Socrates claims that people should avoid things "not required by any natural want." Certainly it is clear that eating animals is a habit we have taken on, but NOT a natural want. Socrates goes on to have the following dialogue with Glaucon:

> **Socrates:** And there will be animals of many other kinds, if people eat them?
> **Glaucon:** Certainly.

> **Socrates:** And living this way we shall have a much greater need of physicians than before?
> **Glaucon:** Much greater.

> **Socrates:** And the country, which was enough to support the original inhabitants will be too small now and not enough?
> **Glaucon:** Quite true.

> **Socrates:** Then a slice of our neighbors land will be wanted by us for pasture and tillage, and they will want a slice of ours, if, like ourselves, they exceed the limit of necessity and give themselves up to the unlimited accumulation of wealth?
> **Glaucon:** That, Socrates, will be inevitable.

> **Socrates:** And so we shall go to war, Glaucon. Shall we not?
> **Glaucon:** Most certainly.

This war that Plato and Socrates had foreseen has been intensely raging in and around us, making victims of all who live in such a numbed-out, violent world. The very food that we are destroying our planet to create is the very food that is ravaging our bodies, destroying our physical health and numbing our abilities to feel. Sleeping humanity has become a growing cancer. Is it any wonder the very societies that are most deadly to the environment experience cancer and disease at such an alarming rate?

As above, so below. We have no regard for nature and, in turn, less regard for ourselves. How can health and harmony exist when we live in such utter ignorance and promote the daily violence against our animals, environment, and starving masses of humanity by purchasing these products of cruelty?

You cannot do wrong without suffering wrong.

—Emerson

For some reason "civilized" humanity believes itself to be above the laws that govern our world. Such arrogance is not held by any indigenous peoples or "uncivilized" tribes. These "backward" people, such as American Indians or Australian Aborigines, could not understand the idea of "owning land" as they felt that they were part of the Earth and that in fact the Earth owned them. Hunting did exist among theses people, but they had great reverence for the animal that gave its life so they could live. They never took more than they needed and always viewed themselves as A PART of creation, NOT the epitome or "Lord of Nature" that modern man deems himself. **When laws are broken, there are penalties to pay.**

These "uncivilized" people, like animals in nature, do not kill out of hatred or try to control, dominate, enslave, or torture other species. They kill for survival and take what is needed; thus, the balance in the natural world is never threatened by their actions. The neurotic behavior of trying to control nature has bred a world with a civilization filled with frightened, desperate, depressed, and insatiable people on the brink of oblivion. You can make a conscious choice to no longer support this cycle of insanity. Remember you are either part of the solution or part of the problem.

Many great teachers have reminded us of our interconnectedness with other beings; yet, few of us ever consider this teaching when sitting down to eat. And **we will**

continue to suffer as we continue to create suffering.
Of course the opposite is a possibility if you choose.

> *The vegetarian movement ought to fill the souls of those who have at heart the realization of God's Kingdom upon earth.*
>
> —Leo Tolstoy

I hope you take some time to give some deep consideration to these issues and join the long list of compassionate and brilliant individuals throughout history who have understood the necessity of nonviolence. I can promise you that the quality of your health will be enhanced dramatically by leaving off the eating of animals, and you will be doing a great service to our planet by doing so and, in turn, a great service to yourself.

> *There was a time, the Golden Age we call it, happy in fruits and herbs when no men tainted their lips with blood, and birds went flying safely through the air, and in the fields rabbits wandered unfrightened, and no fish was ever hooked by its own credulity: All things were free from treachery and fear and cunning and all was peaceful. But some innovator, a good-for-nothing, whoever he was, decided, in envy, that what lions ate was better, stuffed meat into his belly like a furnace, and paved the way for crime. ... One crime leads to another.*
>
> —Pythagoras
> *from Ovid's Metamorphosis*

Gandhi's influence on our global society cannot yet be entirely counted as the ripples of his knowledge, courage, and veracity continue to impact and influence those leaders and followers who strive for decency. From Martin Luther King, Jr. to Nelson Mandela, his words, actions, and being continue to impact all men who search for truth and stand as an eternal example of man's appropriate stature. I find the following excerpt from this great, perceptive, and loving being a wonderful way to sum up this chapter.

A WAY OUT

The following is an excerpt from a speech entitled "The Moral Basis of Vegetarianism" delivered by Gandhi at a Social Meeting organized by the London Vegetarian Society, November 20, 1931.

I used to attend debates that were held between vegetarians. Then vegetarians had a habit of talking of nothing but food and disease. I feel that that is the worst way of going about the business. It is those persons who become vegetarians because they are suffering from some disease or other who largely fall back. I discovered that for remaining staunch to vegetarianism a man requires a moral basis.

For me, that was a great discovery in my search after truth. At an early age, I found that a selfish basis would not serve the purpose of taking a man higher and higher along the paths of evolution. What was required was an altruistic purpose. I found also that several vegetarians found it impossible to remain vegetarians because they had made food a fetish and because they thought that by becoming vegetarians they could eat as much as they liked. Of course those people could not possibly keep their health.

Observing along these lines, I saw that a man should eat sparingly and now and then fast. I discovered that in order to keep health, it was necessary to cut down the quantity of your food, and reduce the number of meals. Became moderate; err on the side of less, rather than on side of more.

What I want to bring to your notice is that vegetarians need to be tolerant if they want to convert others to vegetarianism. Adopt a little humility. We should appeal to the moral sense of the people who do not see eye with us. If a vegetarian became ill, and a doctor prescribed beef tea, then I would not call him a vegetarian. A vegetarian is made of sterner stuff. Why? Because it is for the building of the spirit and not of the body. Therefore vegetarians should have that moral basis—that a man was not born a carnivorous animal, but born to live on the fruits and herbs that the earth grows. If anybody said that I should die if I did not take beef tea or mutton, even on medical

*advice, I would prefer death. That is the basis of my veg-
etarianism.*

*There must be a definite reason for our making that change
in our lives, from our adopting habits and customs dif-
ferently from society, even though sometimes that change
may offend those nearest and dearest to us. Not for the
world should you sacrifice a moral principle. The only
basis for having a vegetarian society and proclaiming a
vegetarian principle is, and must be, a moral one.*

*Therefore, I thought that during the few minutes which I
give myself the privilege of addressing you, I would just
emphasize that moral basis of vegetarianism. And I would
say that I have found from my own experience, and the
experience of thousands of friends and companions, that
they find satisfaction from the moral basis they have cho-
sen for sustaining vegetarianism.*

If you are interested, here is an additional list of reported vegetarians:

ACTORS, PERFORMERS AND TV PERSONALITIES

Gillian Anderson (Actress, *X-Files*), Vegan
Pamela Anderson (Actress, *Baywatch, V.I.P.*)
Richard Bach (Writer)
Alec Baldwin (Actor)
Bob Barker (Host, *The Price is Right*)
Kim Basinger (Actress, *L.A. Confidential*)
Elizabeth Berkley (Actress, *Saved by the Bell*)
Peter Bogdanovich (Director), Vegan
"Downtown" Julie Brown (Former MTV VJ)
Kirk Cameron (Actor, *Growing Pains*)
John Cleese (Actor, *Monty Python, Harry Potter* movies)
James Cromwell (Actor, *L.A. Confidential, Babe*), Vegan
Michael J. Fox (Actor, *Teen Wolf, Back to the Future*)
Jennie Garth (Actress, *Beverly Hills, 90210*), Vegan
Woody Harrelson (Actor, *Cheers, No Country for Old Men*), Vegan
Ashley Judd (Actress, *Double Jeopardy, Where the Heart Is*)
Ricki Lake (Talk show host/actress)

Cloris Leachman (Actress, *Young Frankenstein*)
Tobey Maguire (Actor, *Pleasantville, Spider Man*)
Bill Maguire (Talk show host)
Rue McClanahan (Actress, *The Golden Girls*)
Mary Tyler Moore (Actress, *The Mary Tyler Moore Show*), Pesco-vegetarian
Kevin Nealon (Actor, *Saturday Night Live*), Vegan
Leonard Nimoy (Actor, *Star Trek*)
Leslie Parrish (Actress)
Alexandra Paul (Actress, *Baywatch*)
Joaquin Phoenix (Actor, *Walk the Line, Gladiator*), Vegan
Natalie Portman (Actress, *Star Wars, Garden State*)
Stephanie Powers (Actress, *Hart to Hart*)
Joe Regalbuto (Actor, *Murphy Brown*)
Fred Rogers (Actor, *Mr. Roger's Neighborhood*)
Steven Seagal (Actor, movie director)
Jerry Seinfeld (Comedian, *Seinfeld*)
Alicia Silverstone (Actress, *Clueless, Batman and Robin*), Vegan
Lisa Simpson (character on *The Simpsons*)
Sy Sperling (President of the Hair Club for Men)
Jonathan Taylor Thomas (Actor, *Home Improvement*), Vegan
Vince Vaughn (Actor, *Swingers, Wedding Crashers*)
Kristina Wagner (Actress, *General Hospital*)
Dennis Weaver (Actor, *McCloud*)

SINGERS AND MUSICIANS

Bryan Adams (Singer), Vegan
Jeff Ament (Bassist, Pearl Jam)
Fiona Apple (Singer), Vegan
B52's (The entire band)
Erykah Badu (Singer), Vegan
Joan Baez (Folk singer)
Martin Barre (Singer)
The Beastie Boys (The entire band)
Michael Bolton (Singer/songwriter)
Charlie Burchill (Guitarist, Simple Minds)
Kate Bush (Singer/songwriter)
Montserrat Caballe (Opera singer)

Vivian Cambell (Guitarist, Def Leppard)
Phil Collen (Guitarist, Def Leppard)
Elvis Costello (Singer/musician)
Des'ree (British pop singer)
Bob Dylan (Singer/songwriter)
Earth Crisis (The entire band), Vegan
Melissa Etheridge (Singer/songwriter)
Peter Gabriel (Singer)
Boy George (Singer)
Dizzie Gillespie (Musician)
Dave Goodman (Producer, Sex Pistols), Vegan
Kirk Hammett (Lead Guitarist/songwriter, Metallica)
George Harrison (Former lead guitarist, The Beatles)
Chrissie Hynde (Singer/songwriter, The Pretenders)
Billy Idol (Singer)
Indigo Girls (Amy Ray and Emily Sailors)
LaToya Jackson (Singer)
Michael Jackson (Singer)
Joan Jett (Singer)
Howard Jones (Singer)
Gladys Knight (Singer)
Lenny Kravitz (Singer)
kd lang (Singer), Vegan
John Lennon (Singer/songwriter, The Beatles)
Annie Lennox (Singer, Eurythmics)
Bob Marley (Singer/songwriter)
Ricky Martin (Singer)
Paul McCartney (Singer/musician, The Beatles), Vegan
Linda McCartney (Musician/photographer)
Sarah McLachlan (Singer/songwriter)
Brian May (Guitarist, Queen)
Natalie Merchant (Singer/songwriter)
Moby (Musician/singer/songwriter), Vegan
Alanis Morissette (Singer)
Morrissey (Singer/songwriter, The Smiths)
Larry Mullen Junior (Drummer, U2)
Olivia Newton John (Singer/actress)
Sinéad O'Connor (Singer), Vegan
Yoko Ono (Plastic Ono Band)

Ozzy Osborne (Singer, Black Sabbath)
Steve Perry (Former lead singer, Journey)
Prince – (Singer/songwriter), Vegan
Rikki Rockett (Drummer, Poison), Vegan
Seal (Singer/songwriter)
Siouxsie Sioux (Singer)
Grace Slick (Lead singer, Jefferson Airplane, Jefferson Starship), Vegan
Robert Smith (Lead singer, The Cure), Pesco-vegetarian
The Smiths (The entire band)
Ringo Starr (Drummer, The Beatles) **and his wife, Barbara Bach**
Sting (Singer/songwriter, The Police)
Michael Stipe (Lead singer, REM)
Shania Twain (Singer/songwriter)
Steve Vai (Guitarist)
Eddie Vedder (Lead singer/guitarist, Pearl Jam)
Bill Ward (Drummer, Black Sabbath; Vocalist, Bill WardBand)
Charlie Watts (Drummer, Rolling Stones)
Jane Wiedlin (Guitarist, The Go-Go's)
Alan Wilder (Musician, former member of Depeche Mode)
Vanessa Williams (Actress/singer)
"Weird" Al Yankocic (Singer/songwriter), Vegan
Moon, Ahmet, Diva Zappa (Frank Zappa's children)

STATESMEN AND POLITICIANS

Susan B. Anthony (Leader of Women's Suffrage movement)
Tony Banks MP (U.K Minister for Sport)
Clarissa Barton (Founder, Red Cross, humanitarian)
Yung-fa Chang (Chairman of international business)
Chelsea Clinton (Daughter of former U.S President Bill Clinton)
Mohandas Karamchand Gandhi (Influential Leader)
Dick Gregory (Environmental activist)
Ivan Kostov (Former 46th Prime Minister of the Republic of Bulgaria)
Moritz Leuenberger (Swiss Politician, Lawyer)
Robert Lutz (Vice President of GM Global Product Development)
Howard Lyman (IVU Past President)
Quett Ketumile Joni Masire, GCMG (Former President of the

Republic of Botswana)
Sardar Vallabhbhai Patel (First Home Minister of India), Vegan
P.V. Narasimha Rao (Prime Minister of India 1991-1996)
Sofia of Greece and Denmark (Queen of Spain)
Graham Spencer (Co-founder and chief Technology Officer of Excite, a pioneer company in internet technology and services)

WRITERS

Scott Adams (Cartoonist, *Dilbert*)
Clive Barker (Writer/director)
Dr. Arturo Alvarez Bravo (Writer and pioneer of the alternative and vegetarian medicine in America, founder of various associations)
Berke Breathed (Cartoonist, *Bloom County*, *Outland*)
Rada Krishna Das (Activist)
Dalai Lama of Tibet (Leader of Buddhism)
Stephen Fuchs (Rabbi, lecturer, professor)
Henry Heimlich M.D. (Created Heimlich maneuver)
Krishnamurti Jiddu (Spiritual teacher)
Steven Jobs (Founder/CEO of Apple), Pesco-vegetarian
Anand Krishna (Founder of Meditation)
John McDougall, M.D. (Writer, Medical Director of McDougall Program at St. Helena Hospital and Health Center)
Srinivasa Ramanujan (Respected Indian mathematician)
Jeremy Rifkin (Writer, *Beyond Beef*)
Alice Walker (Writer, *The Color Purple*), Vegan

ATHLETES

Natascha Badmann (Iron lady of Hawaii 1998)
Michael Bennett (World heavyweight amateur boxing champion)
Peter Burwash (Tennis)
Greg Chappell (Former Australian Cricketer), Vegan
Simon Cope (Cyclist)
Robert De Costella (Marathon runner, Australian)
Estelle Gray (Cyclist)
Dr. Ruth Heidrich (Iron woman), Vegan
Thomas Hellriegel (Iron man)
Desmond Howard (Football player, Jackson Jaguars)

Killer Kowalski (Wrestler)

Donnie LaLonde (Former Light Heavyweight Champion of the World)

Tony LaRussa (Manager of the St. Louis Cardinals)

Silken Laumann (Olympic rower)

Carl Lewis (Olympic gold medalist, track and field)

Sixto Linares (24 Hour Triathlon)

Katherine Monbiot (World champion arm wrestler and nutritionist), Vegan

Martina Navratilova (Retired tennis champion)

Chapter 2

——— ❖ ◆ ❖ ———

DAIRY PRODUCTS

How many times have we heard the phrase "Milk is Natural?" That is quite a broad statement. First of all what kind of milk is being considered and, second of all, natural for whom? Certainly dog milk is natural for puppies, cat milk is natural for kittens, and cow milk is natural for calves. It's difficult to argue this fact, as the nursing of these mammals is as natural and instinctive as many act in nature. No sane individual would argue this fact. However, when being told that the milk of a one-thousand-pound animal is a "natural" for human consumption, the true thinker might raise an eyebrow or two.

WE ARE THE ONLY SPECIES ON THE PLANET THAT DRINK THE MILK OF ANOTHER SPECIES.

Imagine if you saw people in a cow pasture drop to their knees and start sucking on a cow's teat. What would your response be? Surprise, shock, disbelief? You might even be disgusted, but pour yourself a glass of the same stuff from a cardboard container and all of a sudden the shock and disgust disappears.

Drinking the milk of this bovine beast is a bizarre and highly unnatural act. What could be more unnatural than this peculiar habit of attempting to nourish ourselves with another species' milk? When you go against the Laws of Nature, you will pay the price.

This corrupt act is made worse by the cooking or "pasteurization" process that all of our dairy products go through. The high temperatures destroy and coagulate most all of the nutrients we might be able to utilize and make this already troublesome food that much more difficult to digest. Of all the unconscious acts we perform against our health and well being, the ingestion of dairy products is right up near the top in terms of disease-producing behaviors.

Cow's milk has a very specific natural function to feed the offspring of these large animals. Calves are usually born at around 50 to 60 pounds. In a month and a half they double in size, and in one year's time they grow to an amazing 1000 pounds or more, nurtured solely on the milk of the mother. This incredible growth spurt is created by the nutrients and hormones in this milk.

DRINKING THE MILK OF A COW IS A BIZARRE ACT.

It is plain to see that milk is the essential food of a mammal's offspring. It is a "natural" in this respect. It is necessary and wholesome and provides newborns with the proper nutrition to build and maintain their bodies without the help of any other food. It is nature's perfect food for the offspring of the designated species. It is important to note that NO FULL-GROWN MAMMAL IN NATURE CONSUMES MILK.

There are no full-grown cows drinking cow's milk. This is another inarguable fact. You cannot find a mature animal in nature trying to suckle its mother. You certainly would spend the rest of your life trying to find a full-grown mammal approaching the mother of another species to drink her milk.

One of our distinct human attributes is the ability to reason. Why would any full-grown, reasonable human being partake in the ingesting of milk designed for the offspring of a completely different species and think it advantageous to their health? The answer is your pick: advertising or brainwashing.

The dairy council is one of more powerful lobbies in Washington and has tremendous influence in setting public policy on Capital Hill. In 1998, the dairy industry spent 190 million dollars on their ubiquitous mustache campaign, paying celebrities and athletes to promote this disease producer. Not only did they get our president to do one of their advertisements, but shockingly, the highest-ranking health official in the land, Donna Shalala, the Secretary of Health and Human Services, appeared with the "milk-stache" in *Health* magazine. That's no different from our Attorney General advertising for the Mafia.

Human babies have the enzymes rennin and lactase in their bodies up until the age of three to four years old. Theses two enzymes are necessary for the digestion of human breast milk. Once the child begins to form teeth, the rennin and lactase are no longer produced, and he or she is weaned and begins to eat solid food, no longer relying on milk. This is nature's plan. Our Dairy Council and "health experts" have different plans.

If the natural hormonal balance in cow's milk, this food we so commonly and thoughtlessly consume, is great enough to support such intense growth spurts for the calf in one year's time, is it possible that this food could be harmful and disease producing in a human body? When a male human being is born at seven to ten pounds and a female human being at only a few pounds lighter, it takes at least eighteen years for them to reach full maturity. This is obvious a totally different growth rate than that of a cow. What problems are created when human beings are fed these daily doses of animal food with all its powerful, bovine-designed hormones?

Putting cow's milk in a human body is no different than putting rocket fuel in your family car; your car is going to have some serious problems running on a fuel designed for a totally different type of machine. The results of both inappropriate fuel choices are disastrous. Our society suffers greatly from this outlandish and accepted practice of feeding on the milk of another species.

There is an enzyme in cow's milk called casein. Casein is used to make one of the strongest wood-bonding glues on the planet. This gooey, sticky substance wreaks havoc in the human digestive tract. It adheres to the walls of the intestinal tract and is unable to be broken down, and hardens, creating a wall of intestinal plaque, which significantly impairs the body's ability to absorb the needed nutrients from other foods we eat. Of course, if your body does not absorb what is needed, your appetite will continue to grow, no matter how much food you ingest. The opposite is also true. If the intestinal tract is clean and the body able to absorb the needed nutrients, very small meals will be incredibly satiating. Ingesting dairy products is one of the most counterproductive things one can do when trying to lose weight.

DAIRY PRODUCTS ARE ONE OF THE MOST DISEASE-PRODUCING FOODS ON THE PLANET.

Because of the large doses of dairy products ingested by our children, their hormonal balance is gravely affected which often leads to what doctors call "behavioral diseases." There are more than three million children in the U.S. taking Ritalin and other brain-numbing, disease-producing drugs, which is a horrifying fact. Many adolescent girls reach puberty prematurely, and a majority of children and teenagers suffer and battle with weight problems and acne due to milk poisoning. Dr. Norman Walker, an advocate of natural living who lived 109 years, did extensive studies on the effects of cow's milk on human glands and found that the thyroid gland can be greatly damaged by the casein found in dairy products.

Millions of children are being dangerously drugged for a condition known as asthma, a condition directly related to dairy products and their clogging, restrictive effects on the lungs and air passages. What a disastrous event to entrap our children in a lifelong dependence on daily drugging, steroids, inhalers, and then give them the crippling news that they have an "incurable" disease. Of course adults are also directly affected by this unnatural feeding; however, a grown man or woman has the opportunity to question and decide for him or herself. Our children are completely dependent on us, and if we have not taken the time to question what we have been told, our children are doomed to a life of disease and pharmaceutical dependency.

Is it possible that the vast influx of foreign hormones we commonly ingest is affecting our glandular system and our hormonal homeostasis? Is it possible that the deep depressions, the emotional instabilities, and the mood swings our society increasingly suffers are related to or even caused by these cow hormones? We have all heard of those who are allergic to cow's milk or who are "lactose intolerant." The fact is **we are ALL allergic to cow's milk.** Some of us just have a more acute response to this human toxin. Of course salesmen have provided us with treatments and products that can help us "overcome and tolerate" our natural intolerance.

Once again industry, ignorant and often greedy "health experts," and hapless celebrities are responsible for promoting the madness that dairy products are "good for you." But we are responsible for believing them. Besides creating an extremely acidic condition in our bodies, clogging arteries, disrupting and impending digestion, weakening bones, wreaking havoc on our hormonal systems, causing painful headaches, earaches, and infections, and contributing to many allergies, cow's milk is a major contributing factor to obesity.

There are more than 65 million people suffering from obesity in this country and hardly a word from the AMA, HMOs, hospitals, or doctors about the heinous effects of this "food."

CALCIUM

We have been told over and over again that dairy products are important to build strong bones and that we need the calcium that dairy products provide. Young and old alike are told this baseless lie, and the belief is so entrenched in our day to day "thinking" that it is a great challenge to find a dairy-free household in this country. If dairy products build strong bones and prevent osteoporosis, why is it that the number one consumer of dairy products, the United States, has the highest rate of osteoporosis? If dairy products prevent osteoporosis and we consume such massive amounts should we not have the strongest, healthiest bones?

Nathan Pritiken did a study on the Bantu tribe of Africa. Hundreds of women who birthed an average of nine babies each and breast-fed them all were found to have NO cases of osteoporosis, and they ingested NO dairy products. They never lost a tooth and rarely broke a bone. The National Dairy Council recommends that we ingest 1200 milligrams a day of calcium. The Bantu's average intake of calcium is 350 milligrams.

Eskimos take in more than 2000 milligrams a day of calcium and suffer from one of the highest rates of osteoporosis in the world. This sad condition has coincided directly with the infection of "civilization" with all its processed, refined foods.

Calcium works as a neutralizing agent in the body, offsetting acid conditions that occur from improper feeding. Many people are suffering from calcium deficiencies because their bodies are in a constant acid state. Thus the body's calcium supply is repeatedly exhausted. **LESS consumption of animal products would increase the availability of calcium in the body.** Once again, a glance over to the natural world shows us that there are no animals in nature with calcium deficiencies. Gorillas, rhinos, horses, oxen, all incredibly powerful animals with huge Herculean bodies, eat nothing but plant life and have the strongest bones on the planet.

A few years ago, I was involved in a motorcycle accident.

I was hit by a car from behind and had my 450-pound motorcycle drop, with the added force of momentum, down on my leg and pin me to the cobblestone street. I was bleeding and in great pain; but despite the force of the direct impact on my leg, there was no break. The ambulance attendants were amazed I was able to walk and were convinced the leg must be broken. It was not.

If you are concerned about getting enough calcium, you will have nothing to worry about if you are eating mostly raw foods. Fruits, green leafy vegetables, seeds, and nuts contain calcium that easily assimilated. Sesame seeds have the highest concentration of calcium of any food. Seaweed such as dulse and kelp are also great sources of calcium. All these foods promote an alkaline, non-acidic state in the body.

In 1983, the *Journal of Clinical Nutrition* did a massive study on the health and bone densities of vegetarians versus meat-eaters. Here are their results:

By the age of 65:

- Meat-eating men had an average 4% more measur able bone loss than vegetarians.
- Meat-eating women had an average 17% more bone loss than vegetarian women.
- Meat-eating women had lost 35% bone mass.

There have yet to be any studies done on the bones of raw foodists, but we can take a look at the animal raw foodists in nature and do our own study. We can see quite clearly that osteoporosis simply does not exist for those that live in accordance with Nature and their natural instincts.

If the information above is not impetus enough for you to stop or at least question ingesting dairy products, maybe the following will provide more compelling evidence.

There are many women in this country who are intimidated into taking artificial hormones upon reaching menopause. Again, the medical message is, "Nature has made a mistake, and we can help you." This time of life has become such a difficulty for women because the body is in such turmoil. Hormonal imbalances are the rule in our society due to our maligned or nonexistent health practices. Uncivilized tribal women and others mammals go through this same change and experience no debilitating upset in their system or loss of bone density.

Many of these hormonal treatments significantly increase the risk of cancer and cause many more problems than the symptoms they mask. If you are concerned about your bone density, weight training is an extremely effective way to maintain or increase your bone density no matter what age you may be. There is no need to bother with any of the hundreds of toxic supplements and calcium drinks (many filled with whey and other industrial wastes) on the market. **Eat according to the Laws of Nature and exercise.**

BGH (BOVINE GROWTH HORMONE)

We have reviewed the massive drugging that farm animals endure as they are fed and injected with antibiotics, steroids, tetracycline, penicillin, and sprayed with insecticides. We have gone over the disgustingly shocking array of feeds that they are forced to ingest, including irradiated sewer sludge. It is no secret that most of these poisons are present in the milk of these abused animals.

Monsanto Corporation, the same people who brought you Agent Orange, the deadly nerve gas used in the Vietnam War, and are now responsible for the introduction of the frightening and apocalyptic technology known as genetically engineered foods, has recently introduced a new product to the American consumers.

Considering that we spend close to fifty million tax payer dollars a year in this country storing excess dairy products that will never be used and literally paying farmers subsidies NOT to produce milk, the need for a substance to make a cow produce more milk is certainly not a priority and plainly unreasonable. Making money, however, can affect reason.

Monsanto has convinced many farmers and corporations of the benefits of having each of their cows produce three to four times as much milk. Money has changed hands, deals have been struck, the FDA, our so-called watchdog agency, approved the use of BGH in 1990, and the madness continues.

According to USDA Agricultural Statistics, in 1960 an average cow produced 3.5 tons of milk per year; in 1990 as hormones and steroids were increasingly introduced, a single cow produced 7.4 tons of milk per year. After FDA approval of BGH, the average cow, in 1995, went on to produce 8.2 tons per year. According to the Associated Press (9/20/96), some BGH-treated cows have gone on to produce 30 tons of milk in one year, more than 10 times their natural capacity.

BGH wreaks havoc on these animals causing their udders to painfully double in size resulting in painful infections and inflammation. According to experts, BGH works like the street drug crack (concentrated cocaine) on a cow. It causes increased heart rate, hypersensitivity, and a tremendous strain on the nervous system. A mature cow weighs anywhere from 1000 to 1200 pounds. If this hormone works like crack on a 1200-pound animal, how does it work on your seven-pound baby? Or a 200-pound man? Or your eight-year-old daughter or son?

In the last ten years we have been increasingly told of a mysterious and new disease called SIDS: Sudden Infant Death Syndrome. Doctors and pediatric experts have continually professed these babies are dying by asphyxiation, choking and suffocating on their blankets and pillows, as if blankets and pillows are a new introduction into an infant's life. Because of these stern warnings to parents to "make your children sleep on their backs," there are a plethora of products and devices on the market to force your child to sleep in unnatural ways. There is no mystery to the rise in infant mortality to those who know of the malefic pharmaceutical cocktail laced with antibiotics, pesticides, and BGH we constantly and unknowingly put in our baby's bottle. Add to this the increasing poisonous and lethal DPT vaccinations regularly administered to newborns that we accept and oversee as traditional medical "solutions."

DAIRY SUBSTITUTES

If you are concerned and panicking over the loss of your beloved milk and ice cream, I have some good news for you. There are some wonderful, easy-to-make substitutes for both of these products.

Almond milk is a wonderfully delicious substitute for cow's milk and takes about thirty seconds to prepare. You need some blanched almonds, a handful or so, and some water in a blender. The more you blend this, the more it looks like milk. If you want, simply use a strainer to remove any nut pulp. It looks like milk but tastes a lot better and is easily digestible and quite nutritious.

For ice cream, you can peel some bananas and put them in the freezer. Once frozen, place them in a food processor, and you will have the richest, sweetest ice cream imaginable. Of course you can add strawberries or blueberries or any other kind of fruit you wish. Try a little raw almond butter or tahini mixed in; it is delicious.

If you love butter, there is not much difference in consistency (plus the benefit of added flavor) when using an avocado instead.

If you are a cheese addict, it is a good bet you are a salt addict as well, as cheese without the added salt is tasteless. There is an inordinate amount of salt contained in all cheeses. Cheese is a densely concentrated dairy product loaded with cholesterol, saturated fat, and the poisonous sodium chloride (salt).

Cheese used to be my favorite food. I included it in most of my meals and actually used to eat bars of mozzarella as snacks. After a year of going without this food, I allowed myself to taste just a bit and really expected to enjoy it. I literally had to spit it out and rinse my mouth repeatedly to prevent myself from gagging. It felt like I had a mouthful of salt and fat. I do not miss it, and neither will you once you reestablish your natural body and allow your taste buds to re-sensitize.

EGGS

What is an egg? It is a putrefied chicken embryo. Of all animal products, eggs have the highest percentage of cholesterol, a fact that the egg producers have taken criminal efforts to hide. In the early seventies the American Heart Association reported on the baneful effects of cholesterol and cited eggs as a food to avoid. The National Commission on Egg Nutrition was formed by these egg-selling companies specifically to challenge these claims. Their organization's name gives the illusion of an impartial government agency, which supposedly gives the facts on eggs. Hardly! The NCEN spent large sums of money advertising in major newspapers stating: "There is absolutely no scientific evidence that eating eggs, even in quantity, will increase the risk of heart attack."

The American Heart Association, armed with all the necessary evidence, claimed that this was "false, deceptive, misleading advertising" and asked the Federal Trade Commission to intervene. After considering the evidence, the FTC filed a formal complaint against the National Commission on Egg Nutrition and its advertising agency. A lengthy court battle ensued, and the NCEN claimed they were exercising their right of "free speech" by advertising the benefits of eggs. The judge did not buy it and ruled that the statements made were "false, misleading, deceptive, and unfair."

Thirty years later these hucksters are still at it, spending millions of dollars "educating the public" and doing studies that "prove" eggs are good for you and "necessary" for your well-being. One of their research tricks is to find people that have extremely high levels of cholesterol to use their studies. When the body is saturated with cholesterol, additional cholesterol is not going to create a significant increase. Measuring the increase of cholesterol after eating an egg in these

individuals produces an insignificant or negligible difference. By seeking out cholesterol-saturated subjects they can
guarantee their studies will get the desired result that eggs
do not "significantly increase blood cholesterol."

The egg producers continue to claim that we need cholesterol in our bodies. This is actually true, but once again
the difference between the cholesterol our cells produce
and the cholesterol found in eggs and animal products is
of a COMPLETELY different nature. There is absolutely NO
need for the human body to seek outside sources of cholesterol. The Task Force to the American Society of Clinical
Nutrition states that "there is no known evidence that low
cholesterol diets are harmful, or that dietary cholesterol is
an essential nutrient in any human condition."

Eggs are extremely acidic and contain large amounts of
sulfur. Sulfur has a pungent odor and has seriously disrup-
tive effects on the digestive system.

The abuse continues in the chicken farms with five to
six chickens living in two-foot-square pens in stacks on top
of one another so they're forced to live in constant filth and
excrement-contaminated quarters. Because they are unable
to move around, their bones become weak and brittle. They
are driven insane by their cramped quarters and the de-
nial of their natural instinct to dust, bathe, and build nests.
They too are exposed to an excess of hormones, antibiotics,
and pesticides. Residues of these substances are extant and
prevalent in the eggs of the tortured beings.

These last two chapters contain all the vital reasons to give
up our animal-based diet. Remember, health does not have
so much to do with what you put into your body compared
to what you do not put in your body. Try a week or two on a
vegan (no animal products) diet and see for yourself if you do
not feel better. The next chapter contains all the knowledge
you will ever need to know about how to feed yourself.

Chapter 3

———— ❧ ————

EATING ACCORDING TO
THE LAWS OF NATURE

It is plain to see that the mass confusion that exists concerning what is the healthiest way to eat continues to grow. Expert after expert comes out with book after book promoting a plethora of treatments and revealing "new" methods and diet plans, including stapling stomachs, "exercise in a bottle," and deadly diet pills. Yet there remain sixty million obese people in this country. America has the largest population of overweight people in the world; 350,000 people have heart by-pass operations every year, 350,000 people die from strokes, and the numbers are climbing much like the number of new drugs that are dispensed year after year. The demand for the new stuff is created by the glaringly obvious, yet often unrecognized, fact that NONE of the old stuff works. When the blind lead the blind both end up in a ditch.

Of course, coming up with an unaffected and unbiased opinion or perspective on the subject of nutrition is close to impossible with the inundation of information and "facts" we are exposed to regarding this subject. Because our eating habits are so emotionally and sensory based ("but it tastes so good"), we are biased, hypersensitive, and threatened by the thought of having our comfort foods taken away from us. The cultural influence that one experiences in this or any civilized country is powerful and ubiquitous. The misinformation concerning human feeding habits is spread by advertising, false beliefs, and cultural folklore. The result is a society steeped in disease and confusion. If we want something newer and better, we must be willing to give up the old.

MOST PEOPLE PREFER THEIR HABITS TO THE TRUTH, EVEN IF THESE HABITS ARE KILLING THEM.

It is difficult to imagine an entirely new way of living. It takes real effort and an adventurous spirit to journey into the unknown and to relinquish the beliefs and habits that have kept us so comfortable. It is scary and unfamiliar to clean off our mental shelves and make room for some new possibilities, but it is also the only way we can grow.

A clear mind and a willingness to be objective are necessary requirements to find some authentic, reliable, and unbiased answers, to the existing confusion concerning proper nutrition.

Nature is a wonderful teacher and always present with her lessons. There is a perpetual cyclical rhythm to our universe that is so beautifully and mysteriously maintained. There is an invisible though constant force at work to keep the planets in their orbit and keep the earth revolving not too fast so as to throw us off but fast enough to keep the sunshine in abundance where it is needed. Animals in nature have built-in instincts and tendencies that keep them alive and flourishing

NATURE NEVER SAYS ONE THING AND WISDOM ANOTHER.

wherever man does not interfere or destroy nature's balance. We too have these built-in programs that were designed to guide us. The problem is that our instincts are buried under a myriad of untruths and misinformation to which we have grown so accustomed that our contact with our instincts has been severely compromised, if not fully erased.

Whether one believes in God or not, it quite difficult to deny that a magnificent intelligence IS at work all around us as well as inside of us. There is an obvious balance to our universe. Why is it then that we human beings suffer so much disease? Could it be that we live unbalanced, inharmonious lives that interrupt and distort nature's intent?

There is a universal organization. Fred Hoyle, the British astronomer and the founder of the Institute for Theoretical Astronomy at Cambridge University, says that the probability of wisps of gas and specks of clay becoming alive is madly improbable and "about as likely as assembling a Boeing 747 by sending a whirling tornado into a junkyard." Humanity is so puffed up with our technological advancements and achievements that we lack the necessary humility to recognize and respect nature's design. The lack of recognition and flagrant disrespect for this organizational force and its incomprehensible wisdom is at the core of our difficulties and confusion.

Nature and the creative energy behind it is ultimately the greatest visible force known to man. There is NOTHING that man can build or produce that nature cannot do away with swiftly and completely. Those that taunt and disrespect nature find this out immediately and often pay with their lives. **Man has a tremendous ego that insists it can overcome nature.** Whether it is building an "unsinkable ship" (*Titanic*) or "earthquake-proof" buildings, devising a pill that will "allow you to go without sleep," creating drugs that will "burn fat" while you lie on your couch, or manufacturing "convenience food" (what is more convenient than a banana, or an apple?). Man's list of attempts to go against nature are long and laughable and the results disastrous. At the same time, by studying and working WITH nature's dynamics, we have been able to build flying machines, automobiles, and many other extraordinary inventions.

The Wright brothers and the earliest designers of avia-tors (including Leonardo Da Vinci) studied diligently the flight of birds and the relationship between the air and wings, including speed, weight, and the properties of lift that already exist in nature. Through this respectful study of nature, they are able to imitate, closely enough, the nec-essary properties needed for flight. Working with Nature's Laws was the only way flight was realized. Such inven-tions, created by the study of nature and natural laws, have provided us with a once unimaginable lifestyle.

Although airplane technology is continually advancing, it is still not as effective as the humming bird's or the eagle's astounding capabilities. Birds rarely crash or fall out of the sky uncontrollably; yet thousands of people die each year in aviation crashes. There is no jet airplane in the world that can drive like a hawk or corner like a sparrow, and there may nev-er be. No matter how sophisticated the plane, every sane pilot in the world recognizes and fully respects nature's force and works *with* the Laws of Nature NOT against them.

Throughout the ages there have been and will contin-ue to be those human beings that contend that they know better and are wiser than nature. They insist on working *against* nature, attempting to dominate and/or control it, and refusing to recognize the inherent wisdom and force of the natural world. Many of these arrogant human be-ings hold positions of respect and are regarded with great esteem. These are the shortsighted "health experts" and "scientists" that insist that nature has made mistakes, and they do a great job convincing uninformed minds that they have improved on nature's ways.

In laboratories stocked with the latest technological ad-vances and measuring devices, scientists insist on taking their lab results and computer readouts as paramount law, ignoring the most simple and obvious facts that are evident in the natural world. *Our society creates havoc by manufactur-*

ing and promoting a toxic diet and then insisting that the answers to the diseases created must be found in a laboratory. This creates the illusion we have today that health is a complicated issue that only can be understood by the select and highly "educated" scientists.

High-tech analysis of the human body and the nutrients and components of our food leads to false assumptions by some scientists that these very components can be manufactured and produced by man and take the place of nature's food. All the while, these scientists ignore the body's ability or inability to digest and assimilate these processed and de-natured products. It is the same as if they decided to use molecules of hydrogen and oxygen separately to water a plant. The plant will die being fed these disparate separated components. Of course, if it is given H20, water, the way nature presents it, the plant will flourish.

NATURE CANNOT BE SURPASSED

Let us remember there is NO confusion in the animal world about what to eat. There are no animals in nature weighing their food or concerning themselves about whether or not they are getting enough protein. There are no animals in nature taking supplements or concerning them selves about their calcium intake. There are no animals in nature eating according to their blood-type. These concerns do not exist simply because these animals are abiding by the Laws of Nature and do not eat according to some institutional guideline, fashionable habit, or for the sake of entertainment.

Indigenous tribes dating back to antiquity have no history of plague or chronic illness. These *uncivilized* tribal people did not experience obesity, heart disease, cancer, "flu season," and the "normal" gamut of pains and infirmities our so-called *civilized* world suffers from every day. For example, the American Indians were an incredibly fit and austere people, highly athletic, and robust. They had a deep reverence for nature, of which they felt a part, and they honored the Earth and the Sun. Then, the *Mayflower* arrived. This boat was filled with people who insisted, as our entire culture does today, that man was made to dominate and rule the world with ideas thought up by man that they insisted *came from God.*

The new foods, all highly refined by human genius, were introduced to the "savage people," including coffee, tea, alcohol, salt, refined sugar, and white flour. Maybe they should have called the ship the *Whiteflour*? By the end of the eighteenth century regular trade was established between the settlers and certain tribes. The new foods were consumed as well as alcohol, referred to as "fire water" by the Indians, and the new diseases appeared amongst the Indians. As the years rolled on, the American Indians were perpetually brutalized and pushed off their lands by rapacious industrialists and the armies they commanded. These once magnificent people were forced onto reservations, and as they continued to take on the "ways of the white-man" their health took a rapid and insidious turn for the worse. Centuries later, these once dynamic and spirited people on the Standard American Diet (S.A.D.) suffer all the indignities and debilitations that our infirm "modern" society endures.

The same example exists for many of the indigenous people of Central America, Caribbean Islands, Hawaiian Islands, and Alaska where health and fitness was the rule until the refined, fried, degenerate foods and drinks were introduced. This phenomenon is already noticeable in Japan and is beginning to invade China, two countries where obesity was scarcely heard of. **There is an obvious and undeniable link between the adulterated diet and disease. The more "Americanized" or "modernized" these people become, the fatter and sicker they get.**

Our national park rangers have turned into the food police doing their best to keep human *food* away from the wildlife, as these products create severe and immediate addictions in the animals that ingest them. Bears will literally rip doors off the cars that contain these heavily processed, sugared and salted *foods*. These animals behave with a violent desperation, driven mad by their unnatural cravings brought on by exposure to these denatured and artificial foodstuffs. One would think if these products cause such bizarre and violent behavior in animals, maybe this is something we should NOT be eating.

Anyone who saw the recent testimony of the tobacco company representatives **swearing** to a congressional committee that the use of tobacco and nicotine was harmless and not addictive will never forget just how willing men are to lie for a dollar. Who did they think they were kidding? Any human being with some sense can easily see the results of tobacco products and the strong addictions they create. No laboratory or scientists are necessary.

Is there any doubt that the soft drinks, candies, breakfast cereals, snacks, etc., that we eat and feed our children, are addictive and incredibly toxic? Rotting teeth and creating millions upon millions of stomach and skin disorders, these *foods* are packed with artificial flavors, colors, preservatives, and substances no human body was meant to digest. Somehow there are no food company representatives called before Congress to explain to our leaders why they consistently create sugar addicts, caffeine addicts, salt addicts, and alcoholics with their "food" products. *Food* companies are responsible for millions of deaths per year and tens of millions of obese citizens; I really do not understand the difference between Phillip Morris and any of these companies that sell such deadly products. Do you?

LIVING IN ACCORDANCE WITH NATURE'S LAWS MAKES SENSE.

"As above, so below" is an ancient philosophical precept that is timeless and precise. Many great minds such as Plato and Pythagoras studied the similarities between man and the cosmos, and the outer world vs. the inner world. In the past fifty or sixty years, quantum physics and the study of astronomy have had a tremendous impact on the way we view the universe. Scientists have recognized the direct correlation between the orbiting planets of our universe and the revolving protons and neutrons of the atom, the prime building block of all matter. Recognizing the relationship between the micro-cosmos and the macro-cosmos is an invaluable key to understanding ourselves and the universe we live in. **The study of our natural world may provide some needed guidance on the issue of nutrition.**

The Earth is covered by more than 70% water. The human body is made up of more than 70% water. Whether animal or planet life, most organic life on Earth has a majority percentage of "organized water" as flesh. *(It is interesting to note the similarities between the shapes of the planets and many of our fruits, all filled with water—oranges, apples, lemons, tomatoes, grapefruits, melons, etc—even a banana looks like the crescent moon. Maybe a universal hint?)* Given the fact that we are made up of mostly water, perhaps it would make sense to eat the foods that are also mostly water.

Notice the difference in texture and appearance of the flesh of a baby and that of an elderly person. You can feel and almost see the amount of water the baby's flesh carries and the obvious dry and brittle qualities of the elderly flesh. This frail bodily condition of the elderly is not the result of the Earth's revolutions around the sun or the time spent on this planet, but the result of years of enduring a cooked, devitalized, toxic diet.

The more water-rich (percentage of water a food contains) a food is, the easier it is to digest. For instance, if you were to eat a piece of watermelon on an empty stomach, your body would be able to digest and assimilate that within a few minutes. However, any processed food from a piece of bread to a candy bar will take hours to digest, and although your body may feel a stimulation effect, the ingestion of this condensed food will place an unnecessary and unnatural strain on the body. This is known as enervation, a depletion of body's nerve energy. We need to understand **that digestion takes a tremendous amount of energy.**

If you need any practical evidence, think back to your last big gathering that involved a big American meat and potatoes meal. Think of the energy in the room before the meal. The noise and clamor makes communication quite difficult. As the meal begins, there is plenty of vociferous conversation, and getting somebody to pass the potatoes requires hand signals. As the meal goes on, the volume of voices and the amount of conversation begins to diminish. By the end of the meal, forks hitting the plate are easy to hear, and people begin to slump in their chairs; there really is not much to discuss anymore. The eating continues, and furtively, under the table, pants are loosened and unbuckled. The announcement is made that "dessert will be served in the den." Uncle Ted is nudged awake as you wonder if you can get to the next room without having to re-buckle your pants. The overstuffed reluctantly arise, calculating the shortest path to the most comfortable chair while calling out, "I'll have the apple pie." Positioning yourself in front of the couch you turn around and calculate the distance between you and the cushions, bend your knees and begin your descent that may be just a little out of control.

You've landed safely, and soon the pie will arrive. You wonder how you're going to "get that pie down" but take comfort in the fact you will not have to move for at least another hour and a half. Thank God for the TV as talking is too much to ask for. Exhaustion has taken over. At least one or two are now out cold, and usually one is comically snoring while others excuse themselves to find empty beds and couches to do some serious sleeping. It will take at least a few cups of coffee for anyone required to drive home.

This comical and quite familiar scene reveals the fact that digestion takes a large amount of energy. Of course, digesting a mass of cooked condensed foods and animal products puts a major strain on the digestive system. What are the repercussions of these daily unnatural feedings? They are many and quite severe. **In fact, it is safe to say that (at least) 90% of our health problems are caused by the deranged and harmful feeding practices that have become part of our daily lives.**

FAT

Obesity, one of this country's most severe health problems and a precursor to heart disease, is caused by putting things into the body that cannot be digested or broken down. The way we get fat is by simply asking too much of our body's digestive capabilities and putting things into our body (in quality and quantity) that cannot be digested. When the body does not have the ability to digest these foods, the body will store what remains undigested as fat. In its intelligence, the body stores the fat as far away from the vital organs as possible in the thighs, belly, chin, back of the arms, etc. As the poor feeding habits continue, the vital organs are eventually affected, heart valves occlude, and acute disease sets in. It is a tremendous strain for the body to pump blood through this inactive tissue (fat), and the added burden to the heart is evident.

It is a ludicrous and distorted idea that low-fat foods such as cheese, ice cream, milk, bacon, bologna, ham, cereals, cookies, yogurt, bread, etc., all of which are heavily processed, will help in the efforts to lose weight. This premise of eating low-fat foods to lose weight is indicative of the confusion and misinformation promoted and extolled by our "experts," and another frightful example of the advice given by doctors and nutritionists.

If you want to lose weight and/or improve your health, your only concern ought to be the DIGESTIBILITY of the foods you eat, NOT the calories or the fat

content. The word *calorie* comes from the word Kilocalorie, which is simply a unit of energy, nothing more or less. **Counting calories is not nearly as important as asking the question "is this meant to be put in a human body?"** If you are serious about losing weight and not gaining it back, this is the first question you will ask yourself before eating anything.

As far as fat goes, there are primarily three different kinds of fat: These three include unsaturated fat, saturated fat, and polyunsaturated fat. The lack of distinction between these different types of fat amongst our dieticians and doctors is a flagrant example of misleading information and abounding ignorance. Talking about fat reduction in the diet without recognizing these essential differences is ludicrous and another example of the thoughtless "science" that is pedaled on a daily basis.

The only fat that belongs in your body is unsaturated fat as is found in such foods as avocados, nuts, and seeds. This fat is easily digestible and utilized by the body as well as necessary for our well-being. Eating this type of fat DOES NOT cause you to be overweight. Saturated fats found in all animal products will clog your arteries, thicken your blood, and wreak havoc on your digestive tract. Polyunsaturated foods are even worse than saturated fats in that they contain hydrogenated oils. Liquids and oils are turned to solids by combining this hydrogenated substance with the liquid. This creates something akin to plastic bubbles, which are undigestible and clog arteries as completely if not more than saturated fat. Once again we find our medical experts and nutritionists have long been promoting low-fat products such as margarine and other hydrogenated foods as tools to "lose weight and reduce the risk of heart disease." These products do the exact opposite, as is evidenced by the ever-increasing occurrence of heart disease and obesity. **There are no obese raw foodists.**

OILS

You do not find oil, canned or bottled, in nature. Many companies swear by the use of the specific oil they may be pedaling and all the health benefits they suggest will be reaped. Flaxseed oil has been held up as a tonic that carries great benefits and will help those who drink it to overcome certain symptoms. The problem is that oils of flaxseed, olives, peanuts, and almonds belong in their respective seed or fruit. When extracted, oxygenation immediately begins to set in and the oils begin to decompose. MOST OF THE OILS WE BUY ARE RANCID. Unless extracted, treated, and bottled with great care, these oils have gone bad and are a burden to our digestion. The very process to extract most oils is destructive to the product.

I once had the opportunity to taste some olive oil pressed in the Italian countryside. It looked quite different from the "extra virgin" oils I had seen before. It was a cloudy substance with a dense viscosity that tasted nothing like the oils I've had in the past. The point is the more processed a food (or oil in this case) is, the more difficult it is to digest.

By their lubricous nature, oils coat the digestive tract and interfere with proper absorption of nutrients and compromise the process of digestion. If you want to use olive oil, do your best to get the least processed oil you can find The oil should be held in a very dark bottle and stored in a cool place and, like ANY food that does not occur in nature, used sparingly.

DRIED FRUIT

Dried fruit, by its chewy and sweet nature is a favorite food amongst those who are making the transition from the SAD. diet to raw foodism. It is a raw food with enzymes intact; however, it has been altered from its original state. Dried fruits obviously have less water in them, and the texture and sugar concentration have undergone significant changes in the drying process. These foods ought to be eaten in moderation as they can create toothaches and the urge to overeat. They also will take much longer to digest than fresh fruit and should be eaten alone. Any sulfured dried fruit should be avoided entirely as sulfur is a known toxin. Be sure to ask your store manager or supplier if your dried fruit contains this deadly preservative. You also may want to try soaking the dried fruit for a couple of hours. This re-hydration process makes the food much easier to chew and digest without losing any of the sweetness.

Remember the body is always doing its best to repair itself and rid itself of poisons, but average Americans poison themselves forty to fifty times a day. Not only do we put such a poor quality of food in our bodies, but the quantity alone is absurd. The idea that we need to eat three meals a day plus snacks is a foolish and unfounded idea that in and of itself causes endless disease. When was the last time you saw a man or woman live to be seventy or eighty who was more than thirty pounds overweight? You do not see this simply because the body cannot maintain its life force carrying this added strain.

There is only so much the human body can endure before it breaks down. So if digestion takes all this energy, and our bodies need energy to detoxify, repair, and maintain themselves, it would make great sense NOT to put unnecessary burdens on our digestive system. We must do our best to "stay out of the way" and allow our bodies to do what needs to be done and this realization brings us to the biggest question:

WHAT IS THE BEST WAY TO FEED OURSELVES?

Under Soul's rule, Prince-Right Eating governs the gustatory estate. Guided by natural attraction, he supplies the right foods possessing all the necessary elements, especially fresh raw fruits and vegetables with natural flavors and undestroyed vitamins.

—Bhagavad Gita

If you were out in the wildness with no restaurants or fast food chains in sight and no refrigerators or "energy" bars in sight, sitting in an orange grove surrounded by wildlife and found yourself hungry, what do you think you would do to satisfy your hunger? Perhaps this is an unfair question that involves speculation for most of us, as few of us are ever in such a natural setting. Nonetheless, would you stare at the rabbits and deer and start drooling, wishing you had the speed to catch them? Would you charge after an animal in hopes of making a kill? Or would you put to use the best instrument ever made for picking and peeling fruits, the human hand? Go ahead, take a good look at your hand, open and close it a few times, check out how well your arm reaches over your head, and notice how well your nails are designed for peeling. What a natural instinct it is for us to want to climb trees, and how well designed we are for that activity. I am guessing you would pick the fruit and not assault any wildlife.

Having this wonderfully fragrant, beautifully colored sphere in your grasp would you begin to peel it and relish its sweet juicy taste, or would you begin to gather some wood and take the time to rub two sticks together long enough to start a fire so you could cook it? These questions obviously do not need answering but nonetheless need to be posed to see our bizarre behavior in a different light.

WE ARE THE ONLY SPECIES ON THE PLANET EATING COOKED FOOD. THERE ARE NO PROVISIONS IN NATURE FOR COOKING.

It is not possible to come up with any truthful evidence to the contrary. These two simple statements are incontrovertible, natural facts, which ought to be testimony to the intent of nature's plan. You can line up one thousand of the most learned, highly educated, credentialed, and renowned men and women of science to contest these facts, and no matter how many scientific studies and laboratory results they produce, no matter how strong the arguments and how many scientific journals and TV newscasts program their findings, no matter what the AMA, FDA, or the NBA says, these two facts are and will forever remain immutable. If we were intended to cook our food, nature would have equipped us with the means to do so. There are no stoves in nature.

There are more than three hundred varieties of fruit of different sizes, shapes, and colors, all with distinct flavors and nuances, ranging from our common fruits of apples, oranges, and bananas to the exotic varieties of durian, jack-fruit, and cherimoya. Botanically speaking, any seed-bearing plant food is classified as a fruit. Cucumbers, tomatoes, peppers, and sometimes avocados, usually referred to as vegetables, are in fact fruits. There is tantamount and clear evidence that the human body is set up for and will thrive on a fruitarian diet. There is no clearer evidence than your own experience.

Eating green leafy vegetables including celery, spinach, lettuce, etc., has become a point of contention amongst certain raw food proponents. Some claim this practice is un-necessary, and others claim it to be vital, while still others will say that vegetables ought to be eaten exclusively. After fifteen years of study, investigation, and experience with myself and others, I have yet to see anyone become ill or suffer ANY detriment to their health from eating raw vegetables. I have noticed that eating raw broccoli or cauliflower can be a little difficult to digest. I have never had difficulty digesting any fruit. My desire and attraction toward fruit seems so natural, and the physical condition of my body and overall health is evidence enough for me that this is the way to go.

There is no doubt that human beings were designed to eat raw plant life. My impression is that eating mostly fruits is the best way to physically nourish our bodies. If you feel like eating raw vegetables, I can see no reason why you should not and would advise that the majority of your intake is fruit. I enjoy a fresh spinach salad every once in a while and have been known to nibble on a carrot or two. (For more on my daily regime refer to Chapter 6 on "Common Questions".)

There is some plant food that you may want to avoid. The simplest way to discern which foods these are is by asking a simple question. Would I eat this food as a meal? For instance, would you sit down and eat nothing but oranges for a meal? Obviously there is no problem with that or with dining on melons, apples, mangos, bananas or pears. Would you sit down to eat nothing but (raw) onions for lunch? Not likely. How about a plate full of raw garlic? It would be less than a pleasant experience and perhaps quite painful. This is the best way to decide what constitutes a whole food and what you should leave alone. Onions, garlic, and scallions all contain mustard oil, which is extremely irritating to the digestive system and simply cannot be utilized by the body. These are irritants that ought to be avoided.

I know that there are many people who claim that garlic has some type of healing or cleansing quality. There is no doubt that ingesting garlic will cause the body to go into an immediate or emergency mode of elimination. To claim that the garlic is "helping" to cleanse the body is the same as pouring acid in your pool to help get rid of the chlorine. You are just creating more problems. A healthy, vital body will convulse at the first taste of raw garlic. The question I always put forth to those proponents of garlic, ginger, or any other herbal treatments is, "What is the cause of the symptoms you are trying to treat?" The next question is "Why not just remove the cause?"

Cooking destroys food. Incinerating your food will obviously render your food useless and completely devoid of nutrition, and you would soon die if forced to eat nothing but the black ashes of food remains. Just as heavy smoke can, within a few minutes, kill an individual forced to inhale it, we also know that smaller doses of smoke over time can also kill. Those who care about their health and their children's health keep themselves and their children clear of smoke as much as possible. There are many new laws being passed to protect the rights of those who wish to keep their lungs clean to protect them from this obvious health hazard. Maybe someday we will realize the health predicaments that cooked foods create. We certainly would not feed our children ashes, just as we would not give them cigarettes. Why would we feed them (or ourselves) cooked foods? Pythagoras and the Pythagoreans understood the benefits of eating "unfired" foods. As his biographer informs us:

> The real reason that he prohibited the eating of our fellow
> ensouled beings was that he wanted to accustom people
> to a contented life so that they should eat unfired (apura)
> food and drink plain water. Hence, they would have sharp
> minds and healthy bodies.

—Diogenes Laertius, VIII 12

ALL COOKED FOOD IS TOXIC

If you were to take a cooked seed and plant it, it would not grow. The life force has been destroyed. A tiny acorn the size of your thumbnail can grow into one of the mightiest trees on Earth because it has this magnificent life force present within its being. Cooking destroys this awesome life force.

Have you noticed how difficult it is to remove the remnants of a cooked meal off a pot or a pan? How we literally need steel pads, various brushes, extremely hot water, and toxic chemicals to cut through the greasy and rock-hard food stuffs. The cooked food has a cement-like stickiness to it that is no less sticky in your body. Have you noticed how severely cooked food can stain clothing? How difficult do you think it is for the body to deal with such a decomposed, devitalized, and denatured product? A bowl used to hold a fruit-salad can be effectively cleaned with a gentle rinse with no "elbow grease." No brushes or steel pads, no scrubbing, or cleaning agents required.

ENZYMES

The human body is not designed to digest dead, devitalized food, and the ingestion of such foodstuffs is a great burden to the system and creates mucus and an acid, a diseased condition in the body. When food is cooked above 130 degrees, ALL the enzymes in that food are destroyed. The destruction of these enzymes begins at approximately 104 degrees. Note that there is not much plant life in the desert where temperatures often reach 120 degrees and higher.

Enzymes are essential to our well-being. They conduct their force through protein molecules and are needed for almost every bodily function. A depletion of these enzymes wreaks havoc on all metabolic, digestive, and assimilative functions, and a body devoid of these enzymes will soon perish. There are four categories of enzymes. *Amylase* breaks down starch; *Cellulase* breaks down cellulose; *Lipase* breaks down fat; *Protease* is responsible for the breakdown of protein. The enzymatic content in a newborn baby is great, while the opposite is true for the commonly sick, elderly men and women of our generation. The reason that high fevers are so dangerous is that enzymes begin to be destroyed at a body temperature of 104 degrees.

PUTTING COOKED FOODS INTO A HUMAN BODY IS BIOLOGICALLY UNSOUND.

Indigenous and exogenous enzymes include those that occur inside the body and those we get from outside (our food). If our diet is devoid of live enzymes, our body is forced to over-utilize its own reserves, taxing the pancreas and intestines to supply more enzymes than they were designed to do. Of course the opposite is true. Eating a diet full of live enzymes creates the ideal situation in which our body's ability to repair and sustain itself is greatly enhanced.

A diet devoid of live enzymes is devastating to our glandular system that is responsible for regulating everything from our blood sugar to our appetite. The thyroid, pituitary, and pancreas are thrown into turmoil by an enzyme-dicient diet, and this is the cause of many diseases from hypoglycemia to diabetes.

CLOSEST TO THE VINE IS DIVINE

ANY type of processing devitalizes live food. Cut an apple and watch how within a minute or two it begins the decomposing process known as oxidation and begins to turn brown. I am not suggesting you throw away all your knives and food processors; I am just making the point that **the less processed a food is, the better it is for you.** If you have ever had the pleasure of eating a ripened fruit freshly picked off the vine, you already know what I am talking about.

It is imperative that fruits (any seed-bearing plant food, including avocados, cucumbers, and tomatoes) be eaten on an empty stomach. The reason is that fruit does not digest in the stomach. It quickly passes through the stomach to digest in the small intestine. If there is a mass of cooked food struggling to break down in the stomach, the fruit will be trapped and end up rotting and putrefying, causing more problems. EAT FRUIT ON AN EMPTY STOMACH. There are many people that claim fruit does not agree with them, and they get upset stomachs when they do eat it. This stems from eating fruit improperly.

It is also nature's requisite that you EAT YOUR FRUIT WHEN IT'S RIPE, AND NOT WHEN IT IS TOO RIPE. Unripened fruit will remain as acid in the body and can burn the stomach lining; whereas, ripe fruit becomes alkaline when mixed with the enzyme ptyalin that is extant in the saliva. If your fruit is too ripe and fermenting, you will smell a hint of alcohol; this means the fruit is overripe and should not be eaten. Our bodies have NO use for fermentation or alcohol and must use vital energy to expurgate the foul substance.

It takes on an average of anywhere from three to eight hours (depending on what was ingested) for the body to digest cooked meals. If you want to make sure you are eating your fruit on an empty stomach, it may be wise to do so in the morning after your body has had at least eight hours of fasting. It is a good idea to see how long you can go into your day without ingesting any cooked foods. You will be surprised by how your body will respond to this change. Work your way up to an entire day, and you will be on your way to transforming your life. Remember there is no faster, more convenient food than fruit.

SUGAR CONFUSION

There are many people who are concerned about the sugar content in fruit. Many who have been diagnosed with hypoglycemia and diabetes are especially concerned. First of all, *comparing the sugar in fruit, fructose, with the processed, refined and cooked sugars found in most other foods is a testament to the ignorance and recklessness of the professionals who do not see the biological, scientific, and logical difference between the two.* Lumping (couldn't help that) refined sugar in with the naturally occurring unprocessed sugars as something to avoid is no different from telling people, "Don't drink water or antifreeze." They are two completely different entities.

Our brains run on glucose. The fructose in fresh fruits is immediately turned into glucose upon entering the digestive system. Refined sugars wreak havoc on a human body, throwing the endocrine system into fits and causing unnatural swings in the body's insulin levels. These abominations create severe mood swings and make addicts out of most who ingest these sugars. Please do not confuse the two. Realize *that there is never a reason to avoid eating our naturally intended diet.* Can you imagine telling a gorilla, "You've got to avoid bananas?" or telling a giraffe "Stay away from the leaves; they're no good for you?"

Fruit is the only karma-less food on the planet where no killing is involved. In nature, when a fruit has ripened, the food falls from the tree. The plant or tree is not injured, and the seeds of the fruit are spread by humans and animals who eat this gift from the gods, securing a procreation of more fruit-bearing trees and plants. Quite a beautiful design. Even when the fruit is picked before ripening, the tree is not harmed, and the fruit continues to ripen and blossom.

It is a testament to Mother Nature's organizational skills that there are hundreds of different varieties of fruit at our disposal. There are all different types of shapes, colors, fragrances, textures, and flavors, an endless and heavenly choice. I do not know anyone, no matter how sickly they are or how deranged and desensitized their taste buds may be who does not like some kind of fruit.

HYPOGLYCEMIA AND DIABETES

The millions of people who have been corralled into believing that the imbalance of their blood sugar levels is some kind of mysterious condition caused by bad luck, genetics, or happenstance, are constantly warned about ingesting their intended natural diet, fruit.

> *Diagnosis is so fraught with the element of uncertainty that no reliance can be placed on it.*
>
> —John Tilden, M.D.

Dr. Tilden practiced medicine for more than fifty years.

There are now more than fifty different symptoms used to diagnose someone as being hypoglycemic. The list of symptoms which includes "mood swings," "headaches that come and go" (are there any headaches that are permanent?), "general fatigue," "difficulty getting up in the morning," "lethargy," and "difficulty concentrating." According to these symptoms our entire population is hypoglycemic. Considering what the average American puts into their bodies on a daily basis there is no way to avoid these symptoms.

The condition called "diabetes," like all other diseases, is caused by putting things into the body that do not belong there. Insulin is responsible for facilitating the movement of glucose to leave the blood and enter the cells. Insulin is also responsible for stimulating the liver and muscle cells to convert glucose into glycogen, which is a carbohydrate and the central storage reserve for utilizable sugar in the body. Whether "Type 1" or "Type 2" (there continues to be mass confusion diagnosing between the two), diabetes is an insulin imbalance caused by a highly processed, cooked food diet that ravages the pancreatic function. The insulin treatments, including cow and pig hormones, given to millions of Americans create what is known in medical parlance as the "latter stages of disease," including poor circulation which can lead to amputation, dangerously high cholesterol, sexual dysfunction, and impaired vision that can lead to complete loss of vision.

This "disease," like all diseases, is caused by putting things into the body that simply do not belong there. *The normalcy of the body is restored by proper living, not by artificially inducing the body to "adjust" to the existing malefic conditions through injections of pharmaceutical hormones. "Recovery" is available for those who wish to recognize the law of cause and effect and change their ways. Of course if your body has become dependent on a certain drug or hormone it would not be wise to just stop the drugging altogether. Take into consideration the intensity and duration of the drugging to which you have exposed yourself and do your best to abide by the Laws of Nature. Remember that a fit body and mind makes the transition from sick to healthy that much easier.*

FOOD COMBINING

There is much confusion about proper food combining. In a world where we literally have thousands of food choices, it is no wonder this has become an issue.

The easiest, most effective and natural way to eat and digest your food is to eat one food at a time. You do not need to have any other evidence than your own experience. Here's an experiment for you: on an empty stomach, eat a certain type of fruit by itself. If you are eating pears, go ahead and have two pears: if you feel like living on the edge, why not a third? Notice your energy level in the next five to thirty minutes; you will experience NO enervation whatsoever. For your next meal have a fruit salad with all your favorite fruits. Mix them all together and enjoy. When you are finished take some time to observe how you feel. You may feel just fine. You may feel a little full or slightly fatigued. Your appetite may have increased. You may notice some slight indigestion, and you will be certain that *eating one food at a time is really the most efficient and effective way to eat. It is nature's suggestion to eat one food at a time*. It might not be the most entertaining way to eat, but look at the mess we have gotten into by eating for entertainment's sake.

Animals in nature have no food combining issues simply because they only eat one food at a time. There are no salad bars in the jungle. If eating a mixture of raw foods is the worst dietary habit you have, and you are experiencing no health difficulties, you need not concern yourself. I do suggest that you take great precaution not to overeat, as mixing foods does enhance one's appetite. Once you have reestablished your natural diet, it would make sense to acclimate yourself to eating at least a meal a day consisting of only one food.

UNFOUNDED FEARS

There are certain raw food proponents that are professing the shortsighted and ridiculous practice that the body is in need of a very specific combination; and an array of certain foods and nutrients, and this requires all types of daily measurements, diagrams (geometric shapes are very popular) and "systems." This practice is absurd, illogical, and completely without foundation. Flying in the face of nature's simplicity, the salesmanship goes on. The message pronounces, "Nature does not understand like I do; you need *my system* to be well." It really is an embarrassing testament to man's egotism and foolishness. This approach creates confusion, undue fear, panic, and worry in those who wish to improve their health.

Remember that there are many well-documented cases of human beings who have gone more than a hundred days without eating (with access to water) and survived. There also have been many reports of human beings that simply do not eat. Most of these reported "breath Arians" are highly spiritual people and live very simple lives. Many of the true religions of antiquity required their devotees to do forty-day fasts, taking only water. The human body has extraordinary wisdom and capabilities if we just would stay out of the way. Our bodies store amino acids and nutrients and can easily go months without taking ANY food.

The idea that you need a certain daily combination of sugars, carbohydrates, fats, or starches is a lie. A clean and healthy body absorbs nutrients so efficiently that surviving on one type of fruit alone is more advantageous than partaking in the morass of poisons the average citizen absorbs at every meal. The human body has extraordinary wisdom and capabilities if we just would stay out of the way.

Do not be fooled. **Your health does not depend so much on what goes into your body or how it goes into your body as it does on what DOES NOT go into your body.** In other words, all we really need to do to return to health is STOP poisoning the body. That is it. There is no need for all the confusion. Health is simple.

Because fruit passes through the stomach and digests in the small intestine, you must EAT FRUIT ON AN EMPTY

STOMACH. Also, you must eat fruit BY ITSELF with no cooked or processed foods. If you are eating a cooked meal it would behoove you to take some measures to aid your body. You can start your meal with a good-sized salad (or a vegetable juice) with plenty of greens to provide you with some exogenous enzymes to help breakdown the devital-ized enzyme-negated food and to help satiate your appe-tite. It is also a good idea to eat no more than one cooked or condensed food at a sitting, as the mixing of cooked foods creates a greater strain on the digestive capacities of the body and has tendency to increase one's appetite.

NUTS

Rich in protein of high biological value, the nut is packed with vitamins and minerals and are quite savory to man's taste. Nuts are rich in starches and sugars and contain far more vitamins than any piece of fruit. Nuts will digest in the stomach and should be eaten alone or perhaps with salad or vegetables.

Of course all nuts should also be eaten raw, unsalted, unsulfured, and unprocessed. Cooked nuts are extremely acidic and the cause of severe indigestion. Sodium chlo-ride, or table salt, is a deadly poison that creates an acid condition in the body.

Obviously nuts are nowhere near as water rich as raw fruits or vegetables. Remembering the fact that the more water-rich a food is the easier it is to digest, we know that seeds and nuts are the most difficult raw food to digest but still easier to digest than ANY cooked foods. I have noticed an increased amount of mucus when eating regular por-tions of nuts. I suggest eating them sparingly. The longer you go on a raw food regime, the less you will desire this type of condensed food. Make sure to take the time to chew this food well to aid digestion. Beware of the tendency to eat handfuls at a time and to swallow the nuts before they are properly chewed.

Some nuts are more nutritious than others. The pecan, almond, coconut, pine nut, Brazil nut, pistachio, and walnut are amongst the best, nutritionally speaking. Make sure not to eat the skin of almonds (you can buy them blanched), as the skin is an astringent and quite irritating to the stomach lining. Brazil nuts are quite oily and may be difficult to digest, depending on your constitution.

Cashews are actually not a nut but a seed of the cashew apple. This seed, unlike any other, grows outside the fruit. The cashew cannot be eaten in its raw state because of the cardol and anacardic; two little known acids that will burn the mouth. The skin must be removed, and the cashew must be lightly heated in order to eat it. In order to increase the digestibility of nuts, try soaking them in water for a couple of hours.

JUICING

Always keep in mind the idea CLOSEST TO THE VINE IS DIVINE and remember that any type of processing will reduce the food's value. However, juicing can provide a wonderful method of resting the digestive tract without fasting. The greatest juicer in the world is our mouth. Its ability, with the help of enzymes in the saliva, to break down and masticate our food, is the first and perhaps the most important stage of food digestion. Chewing your food properly and thoroughly is always a great aid to your body.

Because digestion takes such a large amount of energy, any type of repose or rest will save energy. This energy will be utilized by the body to detoxify and purge itself of poisons. Fresh juices take very little energy to digest, and many nutrients are easily absorbed by the body. It is important to drink the juice slowly and to allow every sip to stay in the mouth for five to ten seconds to let the juice mix with the salivary enzymes.

DO NOT guzzle your juice.

It is also important to drink your juice immediately after

squeezing it, as the breakdown of the food begins as soon as it is extracted. Obviously, AVOID ALL PASTEURIZED JUICES, as pasteurization (a cooking process) destroys food. Fresh fruit juice is acid in the glass, but as soon as it mixes with the enzyme ptyalin in your saliva, it immediately becomes alkaline. On the other hand, ALL pasteurized juices STAY acidic in the body, burn the stomach lining, and help to rot teeth. If you are trying to lose weight and are drinking acid juices you might want to consider the fact that ANY acid condition of an ingredient will cause your body to retain water, causing bloating to offset the acidity.

All cooked foods are unnatural and a burden to the body causing mucus, phlegm, fermentation, acidosis, indigestion, and an endless array of digestive problems from constipation to chronic diarrhea. However, there are some cooked foods that are less harmful than others. Steamed vegetables are the best cooked food as they still retain some of their water. For this reason it is very important that you do not overcook them. After steamed vegetables, there is a big drop off in the digestibility of cooked foods. The less processed a food, the better it is. Tofu, often thought as a "health food," is heavily processed and incredibly difficult to digest. Foods that have been refined, such as white flour, honey, white rice, sugar, salt, and those with chemical additives and preservatives are flat-out dangerous to your well being.

Many people ask if brown rice is a health food. The answer is no. However, eating brown rice is much better than eating white rice, as brown rice is less processed, so at least there is a possibility of absorbing some nutrients. Cooked rice is an extremely sticky substance. So adhesive are its properties that overcooked rice was once used as glue for book bindings.

THE ROAD TO HEAVEN

As we have already established, digesting cooked toxic foods is tremendously enervating to the body and takes away from the body's capacity to detoxify. Eating such an unnatural diet prevents the body from performing its necessary and proper functions. Conversely, eating according to the Laws of Nature will allow your body all the energy required to push out any poisons and useless wastes.

That means that **your body's eliminative powers will increase as you eliminate the counterfeit** *foods.* The increase in nerve energy may cause some acute elimination through the skin, digestive tract, and/or respiratory system. Allowing these eliminations to run their course is necessary and natural. Understanding that the disease (see Chapter 4 on Disease) is literally the way the body restores itself will allow for a relaxed acceptance of this natural process instead of the usual reactive urge to suppress the symptoms with some type of treatment. It is crucial to ALLOW these eliminations to reach completion with no interference.

There is a wonderful saying, "the road to heaven goes straight through hell." Certainly most people do not have to go through "hell," but everyone will experience this certain boost in eliminative power. It may be an outbreak on the skin, an upset stomach, or a series of headaches, nausea, or general fatigue. All of these symptoms are commonplace to those who are making the transition. It is important to rest while going through these eliminations and not to concern yourself about feeling bad or looking bad. You must realize that you are literally ridding yourself of your old body. It is a sort of shedding.

Of course this physical transformation will not occur without some discipline and sacrifice. The laws of the universe dictate that you do not get something for nothing. One of the most difficult aspects of the transition from the SAD diet to nature's way is the sometimes irresistible aroma of cooked foods. Living in restaurant-laden New York City, it is impossible to avoid these sometimes delectable and inviting smells. I have not given up my love for these olfactory delights, but I have come up with a simple and successful strategy to stay with the regime that keeps me feeling so well.

I recognized the mechanical response I had to taking a whiff of some inviting smell and like most creatures immediately wanting to eat the food that I smelled. I then wondered if it was possible to enjoy the smell of these foods without craving or even wanting them; after all, I love the smell of flowers, but never once did the enjoyment of their fragrance make me want to eat them. So I made some determined efforts to no longer associate smells with the desire to eat. This took some effort, but it can be done.

I still love the smell of coffee, still go out of my way to walk down East Sixth Street (Indian restaurant row) to take in the fantastic wafts of cooked herbs and spices, and I am not shy to stand in certain pizzerias ("I'm waiting for a friend," I tell the men behind the counter) to get a good portion of those wonderful nose pleasures. Then I head home to eat some fruit or a salad. You can teach yourself to simply enjoy the smell of foods like you enjoy the smell of flowers—just a little rewiring is necessary.

It is quite common that those who go 100% raw will lose weight VERY quickly. Good news for most, but sometimes alarming for those who are already thin. Most of the time the body will go below its normal body weight sometimes up to ten to twelve pounds before coming back up to its natural intended weight. To many this may be quite alarming, but it is nothing to worry about. If keeping weight on is important to you, I suggest doing some vigorous weight training and or calisthenics to build muscle tissue.

ORGANIC

The general public has been catching on to the extremely dangerous and toxic pesticides, fungicides, and fertilizers corporate farms have been using to spray their crops. Again, man insists on attempting to control nature, and all those who ingest poisonous pesticides are paying a heavy price. Cancer, bone disease, respiratory and neurological failure, and an entire list of other health problems have been caused by exposure to these deadly chemical agents. Once again man's ego has created a devastating problem by working against nature. Some of the richest farmland in the world has been and goes on being destroyed.

There is NO reason for these baneful practices to continue, as there are so many natural farming techniques that not only will preserve the soil but will grow a much more nutritious and tasty product. Organic fruits not only taste MUCH better, but are significantly more nutritious.

Every time you buy a product you are, in effect, voting. Organic produce may be a little more expensive than the poisoned produce, but what would you rather do, spend a little more money, or swallow some carcinogenic nerve gas? These days, at least in major cities, most supermarkets are carrying organic produce. If you live in a smaller town I suggest you organize a food co-op. Co-ops are often successful enough so you can actually pay less for organic produce than you spend for non-organic produce. If everyone decided to buy nothing but organic produce, it would mean an end to the poisonous commercial farming practices. This would translate into less expensive and readily available organic produce for all of us. **Buy organic**. Support the people that support your health and the health of our planet.

You may not always be able to find the organic produce you are looking for and may have to eat the inorganic stuff. I would highly suggest that you avoid eating any inorganic grapes, apples, strawberries, pears, or any other fruits or vegetables where you are forced to eat the skin. Many of these sprays and pesticides are water resistant, and a good washing does not do the job. If you must eat inorganic produce, you would be better off eating those foods that have a peel or a thick skin, such as bananas, avocados, melons, oranges, etc.

To answer the question: what should I eat to attain and maintain my optimum health? *Eat nothing but raw, organic,*

untreated, unprocessed fruits; if you want, you can also have some
vegetables, seeds, and nuts.

I know the feeling that is coming over many of you who are reading this. "Is that it?" "There must be more to it!" "Isn't there some kind of chart I can follow?" "What about getting enough protein?" " How many 'carbs' should I be taking in?" "This just seems too simple." "How do I know that I'm getting enough nutrients?" "My doctor says I can't eat fruit." Ask yourself as honestly as you can, do you *really* want to be healthy, or *do you just enjoy talking about it?* Do you find yourself repeating the lie so often repeated, "I've tried everything and nothing works?" Do you enjoy complaining? Do you like to spend a lot of time trying out every new system introduced? Does all this energy spent distract you and take attention away from what really needs to be addressed? Are you ready to sacrifice your tacit fondness for the confusion, conversations, and drama surrounding your health and nutrition?

Anyone who is fed up with the constant pendulum swings from health to sickness, fat to not-so-fat, and with their physical discomfort will begin to realize that the pleasures and comforts of the sensory world are the **cause** of their problems and will be thrilled to understand that health is, in fact, a very simple subject. Those that do not believe they have the capacity to sacrifice their addictions will deny nature's instructions, make false statements, and continue to relive the same disappointing experiences. You may be gaining some temporary relief along the way only to experience an increased misery down the road.

HEALTH IS NOT COMPLICATED, YOU ARE.

For some people the idea of giving up their present way of living does not seem possible. The insatiable sense of taste is in full command, and no matter how damaging the effects, the possibility of superseding this sense does not seem possible or, for that matter, in the least desirable.

Every religion teaches the concept of faith. To understand what this means requires some mental energy and a desire to question oneself.

What if you *really do not know* what it means to be healthy? Maybe your idea of healthy means simply not being sick, or maybe it means being physically fit (there are many professional athletes with diseased bodies). What if being really healthy provided you with a CONSTANT sense of gratification instead of just a few moments at mealtime? What if regaining your natural birthright, true health, turned out to be the most exciting, freeing event of your entire life? What if really being healthy allowed you to sleep one less hour a night AND provided you with increased energy and vitality?

That would give you back more than fifteen days a year. What could you do with all that time and energy? What would it mean to you to add another ten to fifteen disease-free years onto your life? What would it mean to have faith that there really is a better way to live? What if you decided right now that you are going to find out for yourself if it is true or not? What if you said, "For the next month of my life I am going to do my best to live according to Nature's Laws and see for myself?" Remember you can always go back to your old habits.

It matters little what your present beliefs and imagined capabilities are. You are a living miracle with capabilities unimagined. Do not buy into your past experiences or your present way of thinking and take them for *reality*. You can do better.

Chapter 4

---- • ◆ • ----

WHAT IS DISEASE?

The disease and deformity around us certify the infraction of natural, intellectual, and moral laws, and often violation on violation to breed such compound misery.

—Emerson

Happy is he who has been able to learn the cause of things.

—Virgil

The myths and confusion surrounding disease are rampant and more than obvious to the discerning eye and ear. We continue to live and abide by dark-aged perceptions, diagnoses, and treatments. The illusion of contagion and cures is as fixed in the mind of our culture as the fact that milk is a healthy food that builds strong bones (see Chapter 2 "Dairy Products"). It is obvious by the ever-increasing amount of disease and sickness in our culture that the present paradigm for disease and its treatment is futile and disease-producing in itself and often fatal. We are in this mess because we accept things as they appear to be and do not make the necessary efforts to find out how they really are. Disease, or dis-ease, means just that—the body is not at ease.

Pain is consequent upon violation of the laws of nature.
—Herbert Shelton

The human body is THE most magnificent and glorious invention ever created. It is a self-sustaining machine, independent and perfectly equipped for life on Earth. Seventy-five trillion cells work in unison, all of these cells imbued with an unfathomable intelligence. Everything we need for our health and well being has been provided on our planet, including the proper temperature, the right mixture of gasses in our atmosphere, all the necessary food, plenty of sunshine, and more water than we could ever need. Along with that, we have been provided with natural instincts that are constantly working to keep us safe.

Are you thinking for yourself? Or do you allow certain institutions, authorities, habitual and comfortable practices, cultural influences, and beliefs of the day, to decide what is right and wrong? Is it possible for us to think for ourselves while living in a world where belief systems run so deep in the fabric of our society and daily lives?

In 1634, a man named Galileo was imprisoned for stating with all the necessary evidence that the Earth was not the center of our universe and that our planet does indeed revolve around the Sun. In his time, all of society "knew" that the Earth was the center of the solar system and that was the reality created by ignorant people repeating things that they had heard and putting blind trust in the people they revered as educated and learned. Galileo was charged with heresy. How dare he question what everybody knows?

We can look back and see now that those educated and learned men of the seventeenth century who insisted on their geocentric model of the universe were fools, and quite defensive ones at that. We can also see that when the entire population repeated things that they "knew," in fact they were repeating lies.

The problem was and still is that illusion was mistaken for fact. The illusion that the Sun revolves around the Earth was and is still present. Every day the Sun comes up in the East and sets in the West, giving the appearance that it is revolving around Earth. It appears to be a viable and trustworthy theory and apparently obvious. Things are not always as they seem.

Yes, and today, only a few hundred years later, our society is steeped in a tremendous amount of illusion and lying on many issues. Most people can hear the words and understand **the idea** of living in illusion and see how it might apply to others, but very few are willing to investigate **the fact** that the way we presently view disease is as absurd and illogical as ever. Our beliefs concerning the health and care of the body are dark-aged, superstitious, unscientific, and deadly. The problem is, as it was in the seventeenth century, that we all "know" so much and have an iron-clad trust in our present-day experts.

> *It is better to know and think one does not know, than to not know and think one does.*
>
> —Lao-Tzu

Unfortunately most of us do not know and yet act as if we do. How many of us ever question what we repeat so readily as if it were knowledge? Despite our confidence and comfort in our scientific community, **many of today's beliefs concerning health, disease, and nutrition have *no* validity.** It is important to remember that the power of illusion is great and can be the source of tremendous deception. Repeating things that we have been told, the parrot brain syndrome, is the very thing to create "realities" that have nothing to do with the truth.

Remember this: truth and force have no relation-

ship. Force cannot act upon truth. No matter how many people believe and repeat misinformation, it has no bearing on what is. No matter how many people believed that the Sun revolved around the Earth, the truth remained untouched. No matter how many people believed that the Earth was flat and had "evidence," it was a lie then and a lie now.

Our present day beliefs concerning health and disease are so entrenched in our psyche that a different model is almost impossible to consider, but that is precisely what is quite necessary for those who no longer wish to be confused and afraid when dealing with health issues. Those who are willing to question what we have been told are significantly rewarded and freed from the misunderstandings and delusions so prevalent in today's world.

The following is a different way of viewing the workings of the human body that will provide anyone with the opportunity to see for themselves by experiment and/or reasonable deduction if all this is truthful and logical as well as safe and effective. I am not telling you to *buy my product* or even to take my word for it, but to experiment and see for yourself. It is a wonderful opportunity to gain control of your health no matter your present condition. Do your best to empty your mind of all the things you think you "know" about health and disease. Make some room for some new ways of thinking and remember **that miracles are born of change of perception.**

THE TRUTH WILL SET YOU FREE

This is not a cliché but a wonderful fact that is quite applicable to our physical health. Here we go:

The body is a detoxifying machine. Any matter that is no longer needed or necessary in the body is marked for expulsion and taken out through many different channels. It is a natural event for the body to discard what is no longer needed. The eliminative organs are many: the skin, digestive tract, lungs, lymph system, kidneys, liver, spleen, etc., are always doing their best to keep our bodies clean. Twenty-four hours a day, seven days a week, three hundred and sixty-five days a year, our bodies are responding to whatever conditions to which we are exposed. Eliminating waste and poison is a primary and almost constant function of the human body.

After years of daily poisoning, a body begins to lose eliminative ability and vitality; thus, poison ingested stays in the body for longer periods of time and sometimes just do not get eliminated at all, causing serious illnesses, such as heart disease, tumors, nervous system disorders, and various cancers.

THE MORE VITAL A HUMAN BODY IS, THE GREATER IS ITS ABILITY TO RID ITSELF OF POISONS.

By the way, cancer, or mutated cells, are presented in just about every body. In a healthy organism, white blood cells capture and destroy these mutated cells; however, in a highly toxic body, the mutation is accelerated, and these abnormal cells continue their proliferation. I have seen and continue to see those diagnosed with cancer return their bodies to health (or cure themselves) by abiding by Nature's Laws.

Here is an analogy that might be helpful in understanding how the body works:

Imagine holding a fifty-pound barbell and preparing to press the barbell over your head. The barbell represents toxins that must leave the body; the strength of your muscles represents your body's eliminative vitality. Your body has decided to eliminate some poison and has the needed energy to do so. You begin pushing, and the barbell rising represents a cough or a fever or some other symptom or bodily expulsion. The body is at work expelling poisons. This is good and necessary. Yet we have been taught that this necessary and vital act must be stopped.

A drug is then ingested as "treatment" for the symptom. This is the equivalent of slapping another twenty pounds on the barbell, as all drugs are poisonous and put a dramatic strain on the body. Most of the time your body's eliminative process will shut down upon the introduction of a new poison as it only has so much energy. When the body finds it necessary to do some major cleansing, it may take some larger doses of poisonous drugs and antibiotics to debilitate the body enough to stop the natural eliminative process. The body now uses its energy to deal with this newly introduced poison and abandons the eliminative, cleansing process; so, the barbell drops back down to its starting point. This is easy to demonstrate as everybody has gone through this very experience whether the individual was aware of it or not.

Can you remember the last time you went more than five, six hours or longer without eating? You may start to get a headache, feel faint, light-headed, dizzy, and sometimes even suffer nausea or a fever. Then you remember you have not eaten in a while, so you grab a sandwich, a candy bar, a soda or a cup of coffee. Immediately you feel better and relief has set in. This is a prime example of the body's elimination process being interfered with and shutting down in order to run the digestive system. When sickness comes on, the urge to eat is nullified by the intelligence of the body. The body, in a state of elimination, will cease creating appetitive circumstances until the elimination is complete.

Every morning you have the experience of the body cleansing itself. You wake up in a groggy state with some light-headedness and maybe even dizziness. Your tongue, a common channel of elimination, is coated with a thick white film, your eyes have discharged a crusty substance, and the urge to stay in bed must be overcome by the screaming alarm clock, a shower, a cup of coffee or some other stimulant. The body needs nerve energy to get rid of poisons and keep itself clean. The problem is that in today's world the body is constantly battling to keep up with the endless array of contaminates ingested. When no food is taken in for a certain length of time, the body gains energy and begins elimination. As the body begins its elimination during this non-digestion period, poisons are dumped from the cells into the blood stream in concentrated amounts, resulting in the symptoms listed above.

Despite the fact that this sick feeling is uncomfortable, it is the body's way of cleaning itself out, a vital function for sustaining its health. If we were wise and it were convenient, we would allow these symptoms to continue without interference.

Back to the weights:

As a result of the added twenty pounds of weight (drugs), the barbell drops back down to its original position and must remain there until the body can attain the required energy to push up seventy pounds. The body's intuitive process of elimination ends, and the illusion is created that the drugs have "restored health." The fact is that the body is now carrying more poisons than before and less able to deal with them. This illusion of "drugs that cure" continues to lead us astray and is responsible for the madness and confusion we now live in concerning health and disease.

A vital, healthy baby ingesting any poison, including cow's milk, formula, salted and sugared baby foods, etc., will throw up, if not immediately, within a few minutes. Throwing up and regurgitation requires a lot of energy and vitality. Sadly enough, "burping the baby" has become a ritual of our culture along with colic, ear infections, fevers, and other unnecessary agonies the child suffers.

As the baby continues to be assaulted by these toxins, the vitality of the body continues to drop. Instead of regurgitating and vomiting, the next eliminative channel, requiring less of the body energy, is called into action. Skin rashes and fevers show up as the skin does its best to pour out the poisons poured in. As time goes on, the poor child is "treated" with drugs and pharmaceuticals which are really more poisons and toxins and fed a list of foods to "keep up the child's strength." With such "treatment," vitality is brought to an even lower level as the body struggles to endure the influx of pollutants. As the years go on, the devitalized body's lymph system becomes overloaded (mumps), lungs are immersed in mucus (various coughs, asthma), and the skin breaks out in acute rashes (chicken pox, or more chronically, acne). Allergies, hypoglycemia, diabetes, as well as many behavioral disorders are a common part of all of our lives these days, and all are avoidable and reconcilable.

In today's world, ALL of the body's desperate attempts to purge itself are met with more poisons and "treatments" until the body is inundated with all it can handle and stops eliminating for months, sometimes years, at a time. Then, as we grow older, the onset of acute and intense eliminative efforts of the body known as flu, colds and fevers, and other painful scary events are foisted upon us. These desperate attempts by the body to expel these poisons are continually met by an offensive and debilitating drugging regime that may suppress the symptoms for a short while, creating the illusion that the drugging regime that may suppress the symptoms for a short while, creating the illusion that the drugs work.

The symptoms may periodically end after a few days

of ingesting drugs, and relief from this elimination may end for a while; but not only do the intended poisons to be eliminated remain in the body, more toxins are added. **So the illusion created is quite sinister. We feel better, but the body is in worse condition, enervated and devitalized, unable to push out the accumulated poisons.** Because of this suppression and the increase in toxicity, the body may be unable to do what it must. The patient may feel better, but more serious and intense afflictions are inevitable such as, severe headaches, arthritis, tumors, nervous system disorders, liver failure, kidney failure, skin disease, sexual impotence, heart disease, and cancer.

What many of us view as strength and the ability to tolerate certain bodily abuses, such as binge eating or drinking, smoking, or the ingestion of other toxins, is in fact evidence of a devitalized and weakened body. In fact, anyone who has been abiding by the Laws of Nature for a year or more would be made ill and would most likely vomit upon ingesting many of the foods in which our culture regularly indulges.

Nobody enjoyed their first cigarette. It was a painful experience, and the lungs convulsed and coughed repeatedly to push the smoke out, the eyes burned, and light-headedness and slight to severe nausea set in. As this habit increased and addiction to the stimulants set in, the body's vitality dropped severely, and smoking became first tolerable, then "enjoyable," much like our eating habits.

How many times have we heard the phrase "unexpected death" in reference to individuals who were "never sick?" This means they had lost all eliminative power, and the body's disability to detoxify resulted in death. They appeared "healthy" because the body was too enervated to expel the accumulating toxins. The body can only handle so much poison and still operate. There comes a time where it is simply overwhelmed and loses its force. Medical men refer to this as "heart attack."

To view disease as the cure it is and to stop trying to end symptoms is the only way we have a chance to gain true health instead of living life treating symptom after symptom. Trying to stop disease is like trying to stop a steam engine from giving off steam; it is senseless.

What would happen if you were to stick a potato in your car's muffler and try to drive around? The car would shut down within a minute or two. It is necessary that the wastes be removed from the engine as efficiently and as quickly as possible. When the release of this engine waste is stopped, the car can no longer operate. The vehicle is forced to deal with a substance that cannot be utilized and is poison to its mechanics.

The waste must be eliminated. Engineers and auto mechanics know the importance of allowing waste to leave the machine as efficiently as possible and so design and maintain cars to do just that—eliminate. Here is an entirely new way to view what we call disease:

- **Disease is the way the body takes care of itself.**
- **Disease is the body's way of eliminating and dealing with poisons.**
- **Disease is the cure.**
- **Trying to stop disease is dangerous.**

Not only are these efforts to stop disease dangerous, but they are a complete affront to the laws of physics, logic, mechanics, and nature itself. When the body is purging itself we need to stand aside and let this disease in the body run its course. We need to allow the poisons to leave the body as quickly as the body decides, and stay out of the way. Of course it would make great sense to assess just what it was we put into this machine that did not belong there, and to end practice(s).

STOP THE POISONING!

Now we are getting somewhere.

If you are constantly cold in your new home, would you spend time bundling up and wearing your coat at the dinner table and dressing your family in winter clothes while you lounged around the house? Would you be satisfied that you had the proper gloves and hats and cozy scarves to keep your body's temperature up? Perhaps you could get by, and you could let your friends know that they had to dress accordingly when they came to visit. Maybe for some people this would be a "solution."

THERE ARE NO SHORTCUTS TO HEALTH, BUT THERE ARE MANY SHORTCUTS TO THE GRAVE.

Others might want to investigate to see if there's another alternative, something more practical that might allow you and your family much more comfort and freedom in your home. Would it not make more sense to find out the CAUSE of the chill that blows through your home? Would you not want to check the windows and doors to see if they are closing properly and making sure there is no unwanted air blowing through the cracks? Would you not want to see why your heating system is failing and to check the walls for proper insulation?

THERE IS ONLY ONE CAUSE OF DISEASE. THERE IS ONLY ONE CURE.

Only a fool would neglect getting to the cause of this uncomfortable situation and would continue to spend his time constantly bundled up like an Eskimo in his own home.

One of the great thinkers of our time has a wonderful quote that speaks directly to our society's absurd and dangerous methods of dealing with the sick.

There are thousands hacking at the branches of evil to the one who is hacking at the root.

—Thoreau

Treating the symptoms of disease is a bizarre practice in which our health experts are continually involved. Hacking away at the symptoms is mostly an absurd practice that creates more disease in the body and distracts us from the message our bodies are sending us.

Another confusing, threatening, and errant practice is creating all the new and different names we have for disease. There are only so many ways a body can eliminate, so many ways a body deals with poisoning, and only so many ways that symptoms manifest themselves in a poisoned body. Diseases are named according to what eliminative channel the body uses to expel toxins, the intensity and duration of this expulsion, and/or the consequential effects of the toxins in a body unable to eliminate. There are no "new" symptoms or "new" diseases.

Plato wrote about the extensive jargon used by the physicians of antiquity to describe disease. Through the dialogue between his teacher Socrates and the character Glaucon, Plato scoffs at this nonsense.

Socrates: *Men fill themselves with water and winds as if their bodies were a marsh, compelling the ingenious sons of Asclepius to find more names of diseases, such as flatulence and catarrh; is not this, too, a disgrace?*

Glaucon: *They do certainly give very strange and new fangled names to disease.*

—*The Republic*, Chapter III (405)

If Socrates and Plato were alive today to see the THOUSANDS of newfangled names our doctors have come up with for body eliminations, they would fall over.

The point is that ALL disease is caused by something. If you want to get rid of disease, get rid of the

cause. Do not be fooled by the deceptive diagnostic no-menclature and the *necessary* treatments doctors pre-scribe to scare and frighten you. Understand that there are constant efforts by the medical machine to literally promote new and old diseases to create fear and panic and send people by the thousands to "get tested" for whatever it is they are promoting. STAY HOME. Study the Laws of Nature and begin to abide by them; you will immediately see your body respond once you get out of its way and allow healing to take place instead of trying to gain health by ingesting and injecting poisons.

THE OPPORTUNITY OF ILLNESS

Disease can also be a wonderful, eye-opening, con-sciousness-inducing event. There are a few individuals who choose to view their physical challenges or pres-ent illness as opportunities for self-growth. These heroic souls know that they are never given a problem or challenge without also being given the opportunity to overcome it. The courageous efforts and sacrifices endured to overcome certain situations

WITH EACH ADVERSITY LIES THE SEED OF AN EQUAL OR GREATER BENEFIT.

do nothing but build character in the individual and aid that man or woman in his or her self-evolution. No matter what has happened to us, we ALWAYS have a choice of how we respond.

Some of the most horrible experiences human beings have endured have turned out to be the very thing that gives their life meaning. They discover that the greater the challenge, the greater the opportunity. I have wit-nessed too many miraculous recoveries from all types of "grave "and "hopeless" conditions to believe there is ANY ailment, disease, or physical injury that the human spirit cannot overcome. This indomitable human spirit

combined with the alliance of Nature's Laws is a powerful concoction.

Disease is our body's way of telling us that a severe
imbalance exists. It is a signal that we are living in dis-
harmony and that we need to amend our ways. The idea
the disease is random or contagious is absurd, which
leads us to our next chapter which discusses the myth
of contagion.

Chapter 5

-------- ❖ --------

THE MYTH OF CONTAGION

Gentlemen, ninety-nine out of every hundred medical facts are medical lies; and medical doctrines are, for the most part, stark staring nonsense.

—Professor Gregory, MD

THE GERM THEORY

Bacteria are germs; germs are bacteria, and they are one and the same. According to many anthropological experts, bacteria were the first form of life on our planet. Bacteria are necessary for ALL life on Earth. Our bodies are constantly teeming with millions of bacteria from our digestive tract to our eyebrows. Without these microscopic organisms performing their necessary functions, life is not possible.

Germs are present in all diseased bodies; germs are present in all healthy bodies. When germs are visible in diseased bodies, doctors claim them to be the cause of disease. When disease persists despite heavy drugging, doctors claim that "resistant" strains of these germs have developed, thus insuring a profiteering drug cartel for years to come. If the people believe that there are constantly "new" and "resistant" strains of disease-producing invaders, they will also believe in the need to battle them with the new drugs.

Germs have been shown to be pleomorphic, meaning they change physical characteristics according to their surroundings. Studies have shown that their size, shape, color, and behavior respond directly to their environment.

Most human beings in this *civilized* world have large amounts of undigested, rotting, and fermenting foods in their digestive tracts and have bodies inundated with foreign and poisonous debris, a diseased environment. The bacteria living in such an odious environment are sure to be affected by such corrupt surroundings. The germs proliferate, multiply, and feed on the waste materials, and of course the waste they produce is toxic, as is the food they take in. However, they are not the cause of disease.

If you saw a pile of garbage and many flies and vermin feeding in this pile, would you claim that the flies and rats brought this garbage? The flies and rats are present because the garbage is present; they are not the cause of the garbage. Certain germs or bacteria are thriving because of the filthy environment, but they certainly are not the CAUSE of the filth or the discomfort or the disease that ensues. This fact is so easily and commonly proven by those who are suffering disease and take the proper actions by eliminating the ingestion of all toxins and allowing the body to restore its health and letting the disease run its course with no interference. The result is always the same: health is restored.

At the turn of the century, a German doctor named Robert Koch did extensive studies on "microzyma" germs. At the same time Louis Pasteur had been doing extensive research trying, unsuccessfully, to prove that these micro-organisms were in fact the cause of disease by injecting animals with the so-called "disease producers." Pasteur's experiments failed miserably. Despite the adverse results of his experiments, he *proved* his theories by falsifying and contorting lab results to confirm to his desired outcome, a "scientific" tradition that continues today. There are few men that have done more to set back the health of humanity than Pasteur supported by the experts who continue to espouse and regard his rampant lies. Despite his admitted plagiarisms and fraud, Pasteur is still revered by our confused society as a hero of medicine.

> *This plagiarist (Pasteur) was the most monumental charlatan whose existence is disclosed to us in the entire recorded history of medicine.*
>
> —Dr. M.R. Levenson

Dr. Koch was more interested in finding out the truth than becoming a popular figure. He had great reservations about the idea that microzyma (germs, bacteria) could cause disease. Koch did his own studies and concluded that there were certain Laws of Nature and logic which could not be overlooked. He authored a series of postulates that directly addressed the idea of these presumed causative agents. If a germ were to be declared "the cause of disease," it would have to hold up to the following criteria.

The supposed disease-causing germs must be:

1. Found in every cause of the disease.
2. Never found apart from the disease.
3. Capable of culture outside the body.
4. Capable of producing by injection the same disease as that undergone by the body from which they were taken.

These sensible, logical precepts were, and still are, revered by any **true** scientist or logical thinker although most doctors continue to overlook them, refusing to let truth get in the way of their business. How can one claim that a certain and specific germ is the cause of disease if it's not present in all cases of the disease? How can one claim causation if the germ is present but there is no disease? It is quite common to find those who have tuberculosis germs but not tuberculosis as well as those who have tuberculosis but no tuberculosis germs. The same goes for strep throat, pneumonia, the common cold, flu, and all the other so-called "germ-induced" diseases. Doctors have conveniently come up with notion of "susceptibility" to explain away the obvious incongruities of the germ theory. They claim that a weakened and debilitated body is in fact not disease itself, but just a precursor to ill health and an invitation for the invisible microbe to "take over."

As the years have gone on, less often are germs (bacteria) claimed as the cause of disease. In its place modern medicine has touted the virus as a certain cause of disease.

THE VIRUS MYTH

When Koch's Postulates destroyed the germ myth, the ever-expanding world of medicine and science needed a new culprit for the cause of disease; a new enemy had to be found or created if they were going to continue to sell their drugs. As the years went and medical dominance grew, technological advancements provided a greater capacity for confusion and deception. The pressing need to find a real disease culprit, since the germ theory was incredible, was given a boost by technological advancement and the development of increasingly powerful microscopes. Modern medicine's second declaration of a disease entity was and remains far less credible than their original and, unbelievably, still believed germ fiasco.

Despite the fact that the word "virus" has become

part of our daily lexicon, there are very few people who know anything about this entity. Our culture is once again caught up in the disastrous habit of repeating what we have been told and taking it for the truth. Stevie Wonder said it best, "When you believe in things that you don't understand, then you suffer; superstition ain't the way."

Over the years I have given lectures to thousands of people, and I often ask rooms full of people, "How many people here actually know what a virus is?" This is always a poignant and revealing moment. It is rare that ANYBODY raises his or her hand, and not once, among thousands of people, has one

WISDOM IS THE RECOGNITION OF OUR IGNORANCE.

person been able to give an accurate description of this thing we so readily identify as "the cause of disease." The most common attempt to describe a virus is, "I think it's a tiny germ that takes over a cell."

A virus is anywhere from one-one hundred thousandth to one billionth the size of a cell.

A VIRUS DOES NOT:

- Ingest anything.
- Leave any waste.
- Propel itself in any way.
- Reproduce on its own.
- Show any sign of life.

A virus is inanimate, devoid of any type of capability to act in any manner.

Doctors claim that a virus will "attach itself" to a cell or "inject itself" and then "command the cell to produce more virus until the cell explodes and spreads the virus to other cells." If this were the case, the exponential effect and chain reaction would cause every cell to be overtaken in a very short period of time. That never happens. Is it not odd that our scientists would have us believe that our infinitely intelligent cells would "produce" their natural enemy? Nowhere else in nature does such an abomination occur. **Is there ONE example in nature of ANY species producing another species let alone its natural enemy?** Ever hear of a mouse producing a cat or an antelope producing a lion?

There is no virologist in the world that can prove that a virus is capable of taking any action. If I asked you to believe that a piece of lifeless debris, one one-hundredth thousand to one billionth the size of my body, maybe like a very tiny grain of sand, "attached itself" to me and then "took over" my body and caused serious illness, you might realize that sounds a little more than absurd. Imagine an elephant being "taken over" by a flea, a dead flea, and then the dead flea "commands" the elephant to produce more fleas until the elephant explodes.

Besides Modern Medicine's claims that viruses "inject themselves into cells and take them over," Modern Medicine also endows this lifeless entity with other superman-like qualities asserting that certain viruses are "tricky," "slow," "crafty," "smart," and they can "hide out," "lie dormant," and "gain dominance." If I told you that my chair mugged me, you would think I am losing my mind. Inanimate objects, by definition, cannot act.

All cells have up to 30,000 tiny little organelles within their structure called mitochondria. Inside each of these little organisms (mitochondria) lies a piece of DNA (deoxyribonucleic acid) that is encased in protein shell. On average we lose about 500,000,000 cells per day. There is an enzyme in our bodies called lysosome that helps to break down these dead cells and prepare them for elimination. Other cells commonly use the debris of the dead cells for their own sustenance and through the process of phagocytosis take in parts of the cell, and the rest of the dead cell gets eliminated through the many different channels our bodies use to cleanse itself. What our doctors and scientists refer to as a "virus" is simply this protein-encased piece of DNA. It is cellular debris in various stages of decomposition. **A "virus" is indigenous, organic lifeless, waste material.**

What a tragedy that we have bought into such lunacy and never take the time to question what we have told. Our society is enslaved by this abounding ignorance. We are relegated to abiding in bizarre, unnatural, disease-producing, and often deadly drugging regimes in the effort to maintain or regain our health, depending on a "science" based in psychosis, all because we fail to verify what we have been told.

THE GRAND ILLUSION

> *By closing the eyes and slumbering and consenting to be deceived by shows, men established and confirm their daily life of routine and habit everywhere, which still is built on purely illusory foundations.*

—Thoreau

The myth of contagion is one of medicine's chief foundations, and one of the public's favorite. **Only those that lie to themselves will believe in lies.** Lying to yourself includes being ill-informed or being ignorant or pretending that you "know" because you have heard something repeated so many times. Many people privately embrace the idea that they are not responsible for their health and that they are "susceptible" to the foreign invaders *that take them over.* The tendency we have in our emotional lives to blame others for our unhappiness and to constantly focus and place responsibility for our misery everywhere else but on ourselves is directly reflected in our culture's view of disease.

It is a fascinating study to see how modern medicine chooses to name diseases such as "Russian Flu," "Beijing

Flu" (post Tianamen Square), "German Measles" (if the Communists bugs do not get us, the Nazi bugs will). Its is equally fascinating to notice where diseases supposedly originate; "AIDS" as well as the Ebola virus and the West Nile virus came from deep dark Africa. The subliminal messages are, "You are not responsible for your health because foreigners are," and "Your sickness has nothing to do with your obscene overeating and disregarded for proper feeding." It is quite a comfortable situation to live recklessly with no consideration concerning food choices or lifestyle and have the luxury of blaming our illness on a foreign invader. This refusal to take responsibility for our health makes fertile ground for the seeds of deception. **Most prefer the comfortable to the real.**

Let us take a look at the present illusion of contagion that exists. It is relevant inquiry and not only explainable but verifiable to all who endeavor to learn. We have already discussed the geo-centric illusion created by the Sun rising and setting, creating the visual impression that the Sun revolves around the Earth. There is no doubt that the illusion of contagion is just as powerful.

You may ask, "If contagion does not exist, how do you explain the plague?" Good question. The Black Plague that ravaged Europe's populace in Medieval times appears to be a clear testament in favor of the theory of contagion. Medical experts to this day agree that the plague was spread by "fleas living on the backs of rats." There is another explanation much more feasible and closer to the truth. All disease is caused by poisoning acts; there was no shortage of such behavior in the Dark Ages.

In many European towns and villages filled with the poor and destitute, a stiff tax was charged to those who wanted windows on their dwellings. The result was that many people, sometimes three generations worth, lived in one overcrowded dwelling devoid of sunlight and fresh air, two of our most health-giving natural gifts. It was common to sleep five or six to a bed in these unventilated dwellings. Horse manure was commonly used to stop up any opening where cold air might enter. Fireplaces sucked up the already small supply of air. Superstitions and fears abounded concerning demons, and the human body was looked upon as evil and was denigrated by those who were "godly" men and women. Bathing was not part of any daily regime, and nudity was shameful and scorned. Thus very few citizens ever bathed or allowed the sun on their skin, and physical hygiene was at all-time low. Clothes were rarely if ever changed or washed. It was common for the world-renouncing fanatics of that age to welcome disease as a sign of divine favor and to revel in physical decrepitude. Man tried to immortalize his spirit by maligning his flesh.

There were no sewer systems, and garbage and human waste was commonly dumped in the street, creating a disgusting and foul combination with which citizens were forced to live. So they covered their mouths and noses with thick cloth as they walked along to prevent gagging and nausea. It was common to let the garbage pile up until the narrow corridor-like streets had to be cleared so that horse and pedestrian traffic could resume.

The diet of the day was mostly animal products. Lard (animal fat) pies were common, as they were cheap and readily available. Eating fruits and vegetables was not so common because these foods were thought to be devoid of nutrition. Lead utensils were utilized, and sanitation in food preparation was nonexistent. Oftentimes the water supply consisted of a stagnant moat that surrounded the village; there was no running water.

Due to these filthy living conditions, lymph glands would swell, and the physicians of the day would treat this condition by a "good blood-letting" (which involved opening up a vein and draining large amounts of blood from the patient) or by surgically removing the glands (a common practice of today's modern medicine with tonsils that swell, "overactive" thyroid or a women's breast as a "preventive measure" to avoid breast cancer). These operations and treatments, done in filthy and primitive conditions, obviously did nothing to improve anyone's condition and were the direct cause of many deaths.

ANY society living in this kind of filth and squalor would experience "plague," rat-back fleas or not. The plague ended as entire villages and towns were burned down, many people moved to more rural settings, new architecture was erected, sewer systems were built, and the Renaissance brought with it the beginning of the end to backward thinking and appreciation of humanity, which translated into improved sanitary and social conditions. There was no such thing as vaccines, and **disease disappeared as fast as the filthy living habits did.**

There is no history of plagues from years the 800 BC to 400 AD. The Greeks and the Romans had created extraordinary civilizations that influenced all of western culture. There were public baths in every large city, fresh water, and a large part of the diet was fresh fruit and vegetables. Athletics was a prominent part of the culture, and pride was taken in a fit and vigorous body. Dietetics and private and public hygiene were high on the list of these thriving cultures until gluttony, greed, and corruption befell them.

"What about family members, school children, or office workers that get sick in succession or all at once? Isn't that evidence of contagion?" It certainly appears as if this common occurrence is "evidence" that disease is "caught." Upon closer review, another conclusion is verifiable.

Families living under the same roof are exposed to and partake in the same poisoning acts. These include depending on the same water and air supply as well as the same foods, attitudes, and emotional stresses. By partaking in all these similar or identical activities the chances of similar and common poisonings and body-initiated purging (illness) amongst the family is great. Of course, some family members have more vitality than others, and the effects on each member will vary, causing some to get sick immediately and others a few days later or not at all.

When is "flu season?" It usually starts at the end of November and really hits home by January and February, directly following Thanksgiving, Christmas, Hanukkah, and the New Year. What kind of activities do we partake in? Let's see: There's drinking, emotional turmoil, financial burdens, plenty of gorging and overeating. Couple this with the fact that there is less sunshine in these winter months and less outdoor activity which translates into less fresh air and no sun on the skin plus the emotional dreariness and let-downs of our high expectations for the holidays. The drop in temperature and freezing conditions add to the mix of taxing the body. There are also the inoculations of poisonous and sometimes deadly flu vaccines filled with mercury, aluminum, formaldehyde, and animal puss that our physicians inject us with as a "preventive measure" that add to this recipe for illness that we call "flu season."

There is also the plain fact that there are tacit rewards for being sick. As a child who did not enjoy school, I knew if I could make myself sick, or at least appear to be sick, the reward was great. I got to stay home, watch TV, and get a lot more attention than I normally would. Looking back, I was often surprised that I would **THERE IS SO MUCH POWER IN BELIEF.** actually start to feel ill after acting the part for a certain duration, a testament to the power of thought.

Modern medicine is constantly proving the power of

the mind by doing medical studies with placebos. It is quite common for people to get well, simply because of their faith in the bread or sugar pills that they are given which they believe are medicine. It is quiet clear to any objective observer that people get well *in spite* of their treatments due to their strong beliefs.

Witch doctors in certain indigenous tribes have long performed the ritual of "bone pointing" where the tribe gathers around the witch doctor that spins a bone. Whoever the bone ends up pointing at is believed to be doomed. Because of the strength of the belief amongst the tribe, this individual will actually perish. For a more modern and accessible example, people under hypnosis have actually developed burns and blisters touching an ice cube after the suggestion that the ice is burning hot.

Is it possible that our civilized world can be viewed as a tribe also, and that we are under a sort of hypnosis? Could our own set of belief systems be so embedded in our psyche that we think ourselves sick? When the flu or virus of the season is so prominent in our daily discussions, could our unconscious belief in virus-caused illness itself create disease, especially since there are rewards to be had?

Is there any doubt we would have fewer sick people if companies gave "health days" out to their employees instead of "sick days?" Employees in my company would be told that they are allowed ten days a year to take off to keep themselves healthy, and those that did so and stayed healthy for an entire year would receive a bonus. If companies took on this policy, without any change of diet, the number of sick employees immediately would be halved.

Maybe you know of a person who is constantly complaining and bitter? This person is bound to be a sickly individual and in constant physical turmoil. You may also know a person who is genuinely cheerful and optimistic and notice that this person is full of physical vitality and enthusiasm for life. **Our beliefs and general attitudes are the most powerful factors in the creation of health or disease.**

As with any widespread superstitious belief, our tacit agreement with the germ and virus myth has our entire population living in tremendous fear and has kept the entire world populace unconsciously dependent on the products of the instigators of this deceptive myth. It is rare to find any American family without some type of pharmaceutical dependence and it is just getting worse as the medical machine continues to promote and invent "new" diseases and scare parents into drugging their children and babies as early as possible. "Start them young and early" is no different from the strategies of the tobacco companies and their powerful marketing techniques to teenagers.

If you would like to see for yourself whether or not all of this is true, there is a very simple and scientific test you can conduct. Begin to study and abide by the Laws of Nature and let your body detoxify without interfering. Stop all poisoning acts, keep an exercise regime, feed your mind and heart with loving, life-affirming ideas, and you will experience

THE MEDICAL NOTION OF CONTAGION IS A HAPLESS, WRETCHED LIE.

the health you were intended to live with. You can then hang around all the flu-ridden friends and relatives you want, and you will not be affected. How can I be so sure? Because I have not had "the flu" in fifteen years, and I am commonly in contact with those who are sickly. The same goes for the many people I know who abide by Nature's hygienic Laws. The idea that you could "catch" disease is as absurd as the idea that you could "catch" health. Of course exposing yourself to extreme cold or heat for significant periods of time could cause illness and eventually death.

Here is a wonderful invitation to rid your self of the idea that disease of the body is contagious. You've got nothing to lose but your fear and disease.

Chapter 6

.... ❈ ❖ ❈ ....

FASTING

When animals in nature are sick or injured, they have a natural instinct to abstain from food. This inanition allows the body to utilize ALL its force for the healing required. Even house pets that exist on the destructive cooked food diet have the instinct to avoid food until they are well. It is only we "civilized" human beings who insist on eating while sick in order to, ostensibly, "keep up our strength."

Despite the beliefs of the day, the quickest way to return a human body back to health is to completely allow the body to use all its nerve energy to purge and detoxify itself. This condition is achieved by the cessation of food intake and by drinking only enough water to satisfy thirst. With the discontinuation of feeding, the body will utilize all the fat, bodily excesses, and un-metabolized food the over-burdened digestive tract carries. After an extended period of digestive rest, the unnecessary, superfluous, and toxic matter in the body is broken down, utilized, and expelled, leaving the body in a cleaner, revitalized state. I have repeatedly witnessed significant tumors shrink and disappear during prolonged fasts. A physical "rebirth" is how the results of an extended fast are often described.

In spite of the miraculous claims of certain "cleansing" products and "fasting techniques" there is no more purer, effective, or hygienic approach than a pure fast. The body does not need any help in doing what it knows best. Any kind of stimulant, be it an herb, psyllium husks, intestinal *cleansers*, or oils, is a hindrance to the ultimate goal of a clean body.

Along with the returned elasticity and clarity of skin, finer muscle tone, clearer eyes, and a sharper mind, the increase in energy and ability to assimilate food the way it was meant to be is dramatically heightened by fasting. A certain high is achieved that has nothing to do with stimulation and everything to do with feeling what it is like to live in a properly functioning, detoxified human body. Sadly, this is a state most human beings will never experience due to our constant gluttony and fear of going without food for more than a few hours.

Fasting is NOT starving. The human body uses glucose, complex sugars, and carbohydrates as its initial source of energy. When these sugars are burned up, the body will then begin to burn fat as its subsequent energy source. The last thing a body will use for energy is protein. Most human bodies could easily go thirty or forty days before the body goes into the harmful state of using muscle tissue for its survival. This state of ketosis, the beginning of starvation, is the final attempt of the body to survive by literally digesting itself. There is so much bodily waste and fat tissue on civilized man that it would not be surprising if the average American could easily survive for much longer than forty days without food.

Although the restorative and recuperative powers of a fast are evident and highly regarded by those who understand nature's ways, this rejuvenating effort is highly misunderstood and ignored by our preset day "health" officials. Most of the time it is only the desperately ill that look into nature's cure with any real consideration, as giving up eating is simply not high on the list of viable treatments when in fact it is THE quickest way to return one's health.

Great caution must be taken before engaging in a fast. Fasting will supply all the body's nerve energy to the eliminative organs. In a body that is highly toxic, this could mean danger. Although rare, it is possible for the eliminative organs, such as the kidneys, liver, or lungs, to be overworked, and possibly fail, if the concentration of toxins is too high.

To avoid any serious difficulty, it would make sense to clean your body out gradually for a long duration before beginning a prolonged fast of three or more days. Fat cells contain much more toxin than do muscle or bone cells, so losing weight and being close to, or at, your intended body weight is an ideal way to begin a fast, along with serious consideration of your past and the amount of poisons you have ingested or been exposed to. It is also highly recommended that you get yourself in the best physical condition you can before beginning a fast.

If you have a long history of drugging, whether illicit or prescribed, smoking, drinking or any other type of prolonged poisoning, DO NOT attempt an immediate fast unless you are in a very serious health crisis. Without making fasting out to sound more perilous than it is, I have seen people embark on a fast completely unprepared for the journey with little or no understanding of what is to come and end up in a panic, desperate and confused.

If you fall into the category of a highly toxified individual, you can progressively work your way up to a pure fast. It would make sense to find someone who has experience and expertise in this area to assist you. Before any type of fasting it would make sense to eliminate all poisons in your diet and begin a raw food regime. This will immediately begin to allow the body to start the long process of eliminating without any danger of detoxing too quickly. After establishing your new eating habits for a few weeks, you could invoke a short juice "fast" which involves taking nothing but fresh juices for one or two days at a time.

Any type of fast will initiate body eliminations of different degrees, which may include skin outbreaks, headaches, diarrhea, nausea, fevers, lethargy, or all of the above. It has been said that the road to heaven goes straight through hell. It is very important to have an understanding of the effects of digestive rest (fast) and prepare yourself for the ensuing conditions that may follow.

Make sure that you allow yourself plenty of rest and keep your activities to a minimum. The idea behind fasting keep is to rest not just your digestive system but your entire body. You may have no choice as often times the effects of bodily purging will be physically exhausting. Your attitude and mental approach will play a MAJOR role in how difficult or easy a time you have. UNDERSTANDING how your body will respond and exactly just what is happening while you are fasting is imperative. One thing you can be assured of is that your efforts will bring you closer each day to the miraculous state you were meant to abide in; that state, rarely experienced, is true HEALTH.

It is very common on a prolonged fast to have powerful urges toward certain foods. These addicted responses are brought on by cells releasing certain toxins into the blood stream for elimination. This condition is responsible for bringing on such powerful urges or withdrawal symptoms. Cooked processed foods are extremely addicting. There is also the possibility that after the first day of fasting you literally will not be interested in food; this is always an unexpected and a great help. As your body starts the process of purging itself, the release of appetitive and digestive enzymes will cease completely, so that your interest in food is minimal or nonexistent.

"Fasting to completion," means that your body has been completely purged of toxins and waste. This could take anywhere from five to forty days depending how polluted your body is and how vital your eliminative organs are. You will know when you have fasted to completion by some unmistakable physiological signs.

As you are going through your fast, you may experience a thick white coat forming on the tongue, bad breath, loss of appetite, skin eruptions, and a dark discharge in the urine. When the body is completely cleaned, the tongue will become clear, the breath sweet, the appetite will return, the skin revitalized and the urine will become clear like water. These are the signs your body has completed the cleansing.

Obviously fasting to completion is a major effort that requires a set of circumstances that will allow you to get the proper rest and stay in bed for days at a time, perhaps even weeks, if you are highly toxic. You may have to break your fast before the body has completed its cleansing because of certain lifestyle demands.

Breaking the fast requires great caution. The longer the fast, the more caution is required. Tremendous damage can be done to the body by over-feeding after a prolonged fast. If you have gone for more than five days without food, it is highly recommended that you ingest only a small amount of fresh juice on your first day of eating. It is helpful to dilute the juice with water first, as this will gently bring the body back to its digestive functions. **Your first few meals must be extremely small** and include one highly water-rich fruit, such as watermelon, oranges, or grapefruits. Do not mix any foods after a fast. Do not eat until you are full. Stick to a mono-diet (one food per meal) for at least two or three days. Absolutely no cooked food should be taken for AT LEAST one week following a fast and a minimal portion after that if you must.

As you continue to adapt to your natural way of feeding, the body will become cleaner, more efficient, and will easily adapt to any fasting regime. For years, I have taken on the habit of taking at least one day a week to fast and rest my digestive system. This practice has completely changed my relationship to food. I used to think that food was necessary to keep my energy up. It is now quite clear to me that my energy level is at its peak when taking no food. I can do a vigorous workout for two hours, go through a full day without eating a thing, and feel incredibly energized. I need two hours less sleep on the days that I fast, and any mental exercise is completed with greater efficiency and adeptness.

It does not really make much sense to have the finest car in the world and never clean out the carburetor, change the oil, or replace the oil filter. This type of upkeep is expected and required to keep the machine running the way it was intended. Any sort of negligence toward the machine would noticeably be reflected in its performance. It is the same with a human machine; our bodies need tune-ups also. In fact, given the sorry state of our feeding practices, the man or woman existing on the "civilized" diet requires ten times the amount of care over any automobile. Fasting is a wonderful way to allow the body to tune itself up.

Many people claim that they just do not have the time to lose weight. IT DOES NOT TAKE ANY TIME NOT TO EAT.

Chapter 7

---- ❖ ◆❖◆ ❖ ----

COMMON QUESTIONS

ARE VITAMINS GOOD FOR YOU?

Despite our technological advancements, the human body remains a mystery. There are no scientists who can even begin to explain the force that animates our cells and gives life to this organized accumulation of matter, the human body. We have learned a large amount in the past fifty years, but the present knowledge and understanding of our physical body is very limited at best. In the past twenty years the number of recognizable vitamins in our food and those used by our bodies has tripled. As time goes on, more and more information is gathered and accumulated and the new understandings often contradict the old ones. The *expert* advice of vitamin salesmen continues to change from year to year, so that the expert advice of fives years ago is now deemed obsolete. And the advice of today will be opposed by the same experts who are now so sure of themselves and dispensing that very advice.

As mentioned earlier in this book, it is common practice for our scientists and biochemists to pull apart and isolate certain nutrients in the foods we eat. Why is this being done? First of all, very few people have any understanding of health or healthy practices, and our society LOVES the idea of a quick-fix remedy to solve our problems.

We even make up reasons for eating junk food. Second of all, most of our populace has been convinced or likes to believe that health can be restored by taking the proper pills. Add to the mixture the *health provider's* realization that there are tens of millions of dollars to be made selling vitamins to a shortsighted public. You can bet that wherever and whenever health is lacking, Natural Laws are being ignored. THERE IS NO SUBSTITUTE FOR PROPER FEEDING, just as there is no substitute for exercise or sunshine.

The problem with any vitamin is that little or no consideration has been given to the conditions necessary for its proper assimilation into the body. It is quite clear that vitamins and minerals are absorbed and assimilated into the body in specific combinations. These natural combinations exist in perfect sequence and abundance in nature's fruits, vegetables, seeds, and nuts. To extract one element of a food, highly process it into some type of powder, and imagine its absorption capabilities will be unaffected by its separation is the same thing as imaging you can make a phone call by dialing just one number or bake a cake with one ingredient. Any life force is destroyed by the processing. In addition, it is no secret that many of these vitamin products sit on the shelf for months and sometimes years at a time.

During certain famines, people have attempted to eat the soil in order to stay alive, with the hope that "since plants live off the soil, so maybe we can too." Desperate times call for desperate measures, but obviously human beings or any other mammal cannot survive eating soil. We need the biological synthesis of plants to absorb minerals from the earth and convert them into readily available organic nutrients our bodies can use. The plant's remarkable biological synthesis of minerals is not yet fully understood by our scientists and certainly cannot be reproduced in a laboratory.

Our bodies are made up of iron, phosphorus, iodine, copper, magnesium, etc., the same minerals that are also found in the soil. But **the vitamins and minerals found in the soil are unusable in our bodies; they are inorganic minerals that must be synthesized by plants before being taken into a human body.** Biochemists and vitamin companies refuse to recognize or admit the simple fact that **INORGANIC (un-synthesized) MINERALS ARE UNUSABLE AND TOXIC IN THE BODY.**

Even vitamins and minerals taken from organic sources including plants and animals are vitiated and made unusable by heavy processing and packaging. Many vitamin pills contain refined sugars, salts, gelatins, and artificial sweeteners. The result is that the body, instead of being fed and assisted, is toxified and enervated.

The biochemist looks on all disease or symptoms as a lack of a certain element or elements, ignoring the fact that disease is created by poisoning acts. Even in persons who do lack certain elements, the lack is created by some type of poisoning or unnatural feeding and certainly will not be resolved by ingesting the inorganic elements found in soil.

If you are concerned that you are not getting enough of a certain vitamin, you would be better off finding out what fruit, vegetables, seed, or nut is rich in that particular vitamin, and eat that instead of taking a pill. This way you can be sure that your body has the ability to absorb the nutrients the way nature intended. Remember that our bodies need so little food and that deficiencies only will occur if you refuse to recognize your biological set and defile the body with pharmaceuticals and/or poor grade foods and drinks.

WHAT ABOUT HERBS?

Echinacea, golden seal, various roots, and many other herbs have gained tremendous popularity in the past ten years. I am thankful to see that there are millions of people recognizing the poisonous nature and deadly "side effects" of the drugs the pharmaceutical companies continue to peddle. According to the *Wall Street Journal*, there are "128,000 deaths a year from improperly taken prescription drugs." I wonder how many deaths there are from properly taken prescription drugs.

It is great that people are looking to the alternative methods for the treatment of disease. Despite all the hype over herbal remedies, the wise man or woman will realize that **there really is no shortcut or alternative to health; you either practice health or you do not.**

The essential message of this book is that ALL disease is caused by something, and the only real solution is to get to the root of the problem and eliminate it. IF THERE IS NO CAUSE OF DISEASE, THERE WILL BE NO SYMPTOMS OF DISEASE. Herbs are given as remedies to alleviate certain symptoms. They have a stimulating effect on the body and cause certain organs to go into a state of rapid elimination due to the irritation the herbs cause. This is quite enervating to your body and each time an organ is artificially stimulated or poisoned, it loses some of its inherited efficacy. There is no such thing as a free lunch in the physical world; you don't get something for nothing. With each stimulation, the body loses some natural force.

For instance, the narcotic caffeine found in coffee, tea, and soda will send a surge of energy through the body while in the blood stream; however, when the buzz is over, the body's available energy falls proportionately as low as it was high. The price you pay for this high is an extremely disrupted digestive system, an acid condition in the stomach, and with continued use, a need for an addiction to the drug caffeine. Drinking alcohol is a seemingly wonderful way to forget all your problems and relax your body. The problem is that when you wake up the next day, your difficulties are still staring you in the face, and your body is worse off than when you first decided upon your "solution."

If you are suffering from a severe headache or from some

other type of malady and what you desire is instant relief, as a rule you would be much better off taking an herb than a drug. There is nothing wrong with trying to gain a little relief, but **do not fool yourself into thinking that relief has anything to do with being healthy.** Please do yourself a favor and do not rely on any type of herb or supplement for your well-being.

SHOULD I DRINK A LOT OF WATER?

There is a common belief that drinking six to eight glasses of water a day is a healthy practice and that flushing out the body is beneficial. This is a myth created by misunderstanding. First of all, why does your body need to be flushed out, and second of all, just what is it you are flushing?

Hydropathy, or the "water cure," was utilized by the original hygienists. Dr. Sylvester Graham, Dr. Russell Trall, Dr. Issac Jennings, and Dr. George Field all utilized this technique in healing their sick patients. The program, originated in nature and practiced by all sick and injured animals, consists of taking no food plus drinking water to satisfy any thirst and keep the eliminative organs running. This is called FASTING and is THE most effective way to return a body to health. When taking no food, we should drink small amounts of water. Because of cessation of eating and the absence of water obtained through fruits and vegetables, our bodies are in need of water.

The point that needs to be clarified is that **it is not the water that makes a body well, but the cessation of food and purging of poisons that inevitably takes place when the digestive system is resting.** To reiterate, when the digestive system is at rest, the eliminative organs utilize the unused nerve energy to clean the body. The water taken during a fast is simply a way to allow the body to operate without ingesting and digesting any food. The water is not healing, curing, or flushing; it is simply aiding the body in its efforts to restore order and well being.

Of course these doctors and patients experienced tremendous success in allowing the body to heal itself as the body is quite good at it, but for the past hundred years or more, the misunderstanding that water is a curative agent has grown to become another "reality" that has little to do with the truth. The absurdity that water is some type of health tonic with healing powers is ridiculous.

Drinking large amounts of water is not a healthy practice, puts undue strain on the kidneys, and can cause kidney stones. It is also important not to drink water while eating as the water can negate enzyme activity and disturb the digestive process. If you are eating mostly raw foods you will never have to concern yourself about water intake as most fruits and vegetables are made up entirely of water.

One of the most horrendous crimes against the unknowing public is the lethal array of toxins commonly dumped into our water supplies. Chlorine was one of the first chemical weapons ever used in war (World War I) to burn out the guts of the enemy. It is a highly toxic anti-biological substance put in water ostensibly for our *protection* against bacteria.

Fluoride, an aluminum by-product, is the number one ingredient in rat poison. If you have any doubt about the toxicity of fluoride, you can take a look at the large container of fluoride your dentist has in his office and you will see quite clearly the international sign for poison, the skull and cross bones. Not only does fluoride not keep your teeth strong, it will destroy them and your bones. According to Dr. Dean Burke at the National Cancer Institute, more than 60,000 people each year succumb to the cancer caused by ingesting this crippling toxin. Read Dr. John Yiamouyiannis' book *Fluoride the Aging Factor* to find out more about the treachery of this industrial waste pawned off as a health elixir.

The cleanest water on the planet is steam distilled water. Avoid chemically distilled water and be wary of mineral water, as some contain inorganic compounds. For washing your fruits and vegetables, it would make great sense to buy a high-quality water purifier. There are many on the market that can take at least 90% of the chlorine out as well as remove a large amount of heavy metals.

Some states allow as much as 49% of tap water to be mixed in with the bottled water, without having to inform the buyer. Tap water is filled with many other toxins and industrial wastes other than fluoride and chlorine, including lead and many inorganic compounds. If you are serious about your health, you will avoid tap water at all costs.

IS THE SUN BAD FOR YOU?

Claiming that the "sun causes cancer" is the same as saying that "water causes drowning." Without the sun there would simply be no life on this planet. The places on the globe where the sun shines the most are the very places where the most rich and profound vegetation and life exists. The closer to the equator one travels, the more abundant the greenery. Not much grows in the polar regions, and there are only a select few species that exist in these sun-deprived locations. Most plants and vegetation simply cannot survive without the sun. The sun is necessary for our health. Those that avoid the sun entirely are asking for trouble.

There are certain natural, biological necessities for life such as air, water, food, and sunshine. What would you tell someone who told you to "stay away from the air?" Certainly the sun can damage your skin if you repeatedly overexpose yourself and allow yourself to be burned. Sticking your head in a pail of water for a couple of minutes could be damaging to your health as well, for that matter. The blanket statements made by our health officials to "stay out of the sun" are a good indication of the insanity that runs rampant in the "health" field.

If you have extremely light skin, you obviously must take some extra caution. It would make sense for you to only go in the sun early or late in the day when the suns rays are less potent. Pay attention to how your skin feels and if you experience a burning sensation, get into some shade or cover yourself up. Your body will tell you when you have had enough sun; all you have to do is pay attention.

Eating according to the Laws of Nature will also provide your skin with tremendous advantage that cannot be acquired from any lotion or sun block. I noticed a dramatic difference in the quality and resilience of my skin once I began to abide by the Laws of Nature. You will too.

It is a good idea to get as much of your skin exposed to the sun as possible, especially if your lifestyle does not allow much time in the outdoors. Most people in civilized society are constantly clothed and indoors for weeks, months, and sometimes years at a time. This is an extremely unhealthy way to live. If you work in an office, make it a point to get yourself outside and expose your skin to the sun as often as you can. Even if you live in a cold climate, you must make the effort to sun yourself on a regular basis, if only for five or ten minutes at a time.

Even during the coldest months of the year, there are days when the **sun is shining and the wind is still,** and I am able to get some exposure to the sun without getting cold at all. I often find myself in the park exercising in the dead of winter, stripping off layer after layer until I am shirtless and sometimes down to my shorts. I actually find I am not only comfortable, but I actually break a sweat while the sun shines on my skin. This is incredibly invigorating, and I find I feel quite revitalized and spirited after these sessions. Be wary of over exposure to frigid temperatures, as such exposure is enervating and can cause illness.

Nude sunbathing is recommended, but unfortunately our prudish society frowns upon such a practice. Nonetheless it is very good idea to allow the sun to shine on your entire body even if only for a few minutes.

Stay away from all sun blocks and chemical products, as

they are pointless and dangerous. When you are in the sun, your skin pores open up and take in these chemical agents and toxins. If you are concerned about sun damage to your skin, simply be reasonable and limit your exposure.

WHAT DO *YOU* EAT?

This really does not matter. What I eat has no bearing on what the Laws of Nature proclaim. If I ate steak with chocolate sauce and chased it with bourbon for every meal, it would not take away from the truth of how human beings were meant to nourish themselves, or from the truth of the knowledge you find in this book. If I decide one day that I want to include cooked foods in my regime, it would not change the natural facts. The point is that **personal habits and preferences do not affect what is law.** I preface this section with these statements because I have seen and continue to see and hear people who claim to have some *special insight* and create their own personalized *versions* of Nature's Laws to either suite their taste buds and lifestyles or their pocket books.

Nonetheless I understand the genuine interest of those who are looking to make this transition, so here it is. I eat nothing but sun-cooked, raw food. And a normal day of eating might look like this:

BREAKFAST

I do not eat breakfast or take ANY food (or juice) before noon.

LUNCH

My first meal of the day (around 1 or 2 PM) usually consists of the tastiest fruits available, such as (in order of preference): Mangoes, oranges, pears, and/or grapefruit. I'll try to eat only one type of these fruits and may eat two or four of them, depending how hungry I may be. If I am not quite satiated I may add a couple of bananas and/or avocados.

SNACKS

Bananas, avocados, oranges, apples, raw unsalted nuts or seeds.

DINNER

The biggest meal of my day, my dinner consists of a large salad.

The ingredients are:

Avocado (1 or 2), Tomatoes (2 or 3), Cucumber (1), Sprouts (alfalfa, onion, etc.), and Dulse Seaweed. It is absolutely delicious. (See Neat Things to Eat for a more complete recipe.)

Some additional options for this salad include pears, apples, zucchini, spinach, dulse leafs, sunflower seeds, raisins, chives (an herb, but quite mild), lemon juice, orange juice, grapefruit, or a mixture. Try throwing a mango in the blender with orange and lemon juice for an exquisite dressing! Stay clear of vinegar as it is a ferment and will completely disrupt the digestion process and cause other foods in the stomach to turn bad.

Once a week I take a day off from eating for at least twenty-four hours. Eating so simply affords me a lot of extra time throughout my day. Unlike most people of our culture, I am not bound by meal times or the enslaving urge to not miss a meal. The idea that human beings need to eat three meals a day plus snacks is just not true. This overfeeding is a form of comfort, is an addiction, and is in fact, a major cause of disease.

Eating according to the Laws of Nature and **not** the laws of culture will create a significant amount of freedom in many areas of your life, as any simplifying efforts usually do. Eating in this manner you will begin to catch a glimpse of the wasted time spent thinking about, planning for, preparing, and cleaning up after our meals as well as all the time spent recovering from them in sickness. What a tremendous gift to find a simpler way to live that will provide some space in your life.

Chapter 8

······· * ◆ * ·······

NEAT THINGS TO EAT

Here are some suggestions for those who are interested in making these new food choices and might want a few examples of what it looks like to eat raw food. If you plan to make the change, it is vital that you keep your kitchen counter stocked with your favorite fresh produce. I also suggested getting rid of all your "non-foods" to make room for the new.

Remember to buy organic and to make sure your fruit is always ripe and not too ripe. As a rule it is NOT a good idea to refrigerate your fruit unless it is in danger of becoming overripe. In a short time you will become an expert at picking fruits and vegetables. For now, it is a good idea to seek out your local green grocer to ask for tips on picking the best produce. Remember, there more than three hundred varieties of different fruits! Be adventurous and try some things your old self would usually avoid.

As far as equipment goes, you may want to invest in an electric citrus juicer, that will make orange, grape-fruit, and lemon juice very quickly. I have used the one made by the Braun company, and I am very happy with it as it is relatively cheap, works great, and takes just a few minutes to clean. Of course you could just use a regular old hand juicer if you want to keep your equipment really simple. If you expect the transition to the natural diet to be difficult, or if you just want to increase your food choices, you may want to invest in a vegetable juicer. There are so many on the market now so it is hard to say which one is best. I will say that for the past twenty years or so I have not heard one complaint from the many people who have been using the Champion juicer. This juicer can make every vegetable juice AND turn any nut into freshly made nut butters, which are quite delicious. This juicer is extremely durable and will last forever. Make sure you have a blender, and you may want to invest in food processor.

BREAKFAST

It is NOT the most important meal of the day. My suggestion is to keep it light and simple or just skip it altogether. You can get very used to not eating until noon after just a few days of self-discipline. You should avoid eating any condensed foods such as dried fruit, seeds, or nuts and try not to mix anything.

- Fresh Orange Juice
- Fresh Grapefruit Juice
- Fresh Apple Juice
- Cantaloupe
- Bananas
- Mango
- Peaches
- Pears
- Strawberries
- Blueberries
- Nectarines
- Watermelon

LUNCH

Quick Stuff:

- Avocado
- Honeydew melon
- Sunflower seeds and Raisins
- Macadamia nuts
- Bananas
- Grapes
- Oranges
- Cashews
- Dried fruit, seeds, and nuts
- Design your own trail mix
- Carrot juice mixed with apples and/or celery, spinach, and/or beets
- Melon (you pick) and a banana in a blender –SSSSMOOOTHIE!
- Almond milk: put a handful of blanched almonds in a blender with 10 to 12 ounces of water. Try mixing in a banana or a pear!

Not So Quick:

Mango salad
Mesculin greens, sliced mango, raisins, carrots, and sunflower seeds. Add lemon, orange, or grapefruit juice for dressing.

Gazpacho soup
In a blender put tomatoes, cucumber, lemon juice, fresh corn, basil, and scallions (optioal). Mix. Do not over-blend as this will destroy the chunky texture. Try refrigerating for added refreshment.

If you are in an office job and do not have a lot of time for your meals, it is no problem since eating raw is the easiest way to go. There is nothing quicker or more convenient than an apple, orange, banana, bag of nuts, or raisins. A cantaloupe or honeydew melon is an entire meal that comes with its own built-in bowl. It is helpful to carry around a good-sized pocket knife with a stainless steel blade to cut your fruit.

If you have a business lunch, you can call ahead to make sure they can prepare a salad for you. It is always a good idea to eat before you show up so that you are less tempted to eat something you did not plan to eat.

DINNER

Casaba melon
Or any other melon with lime juice.

Guacamole
Chopped avocados, tomatoes, lemon and/or lime juice, and chives. Chop up some cucumber, carrots, zucchini, and celery for dipping.

Matt's Salad
A handful of dulse (seaweed) leaves marinated for 5 minutes underneath 3 chopped tomatoes, 2 chopped avocado, 1 chopped cucumber (I prefer kirby), a garden blend of sprouts (alfalfa, onion, clover, etc), and some dulse flakes sprinkled on top. I also enjoy some raw corn in this concoction occasionally.

Tomato sauce
Soak a handful of large, pitted dates (about 12) and a large handful of dried tomatoes in purified water for 2 to 3 hours. Place in a blender or food processor with 3 or 4 chopped, ripe tomatoes and a chopped stalk of celery. Blend until thoroughly mixed. You can cut open avocados and place a dollop of this tomato sauce on either half. Really delicious!

Cuke Salad

Diced cucumbers and tomatoes with dill and lemon juice.

Fruit Salad

Diced mangos, bananas, raisins, and coconut flakes.

DESSERT

Ice Cream:

If you want a great desert, try freezing peeled ripe bananas, and putting them in a food processor. You can add a little raw almond butter or tahini (raw ground sesame seeds) as well as some strawberries or blueberries.

Apple pie:

Crust: Soak a large handful (12 to 15) of pitted dates in purified water for 2 to 3 hours. Drain and put the soaked dates in the food processor. Add about 8 ounces of walnuts and/or pecans and about 8 ounces of sunflower seeds. Mix until they become a thick paste. This is your pie crust that you will spread evenly into your pie dish. It is fine if there are small chunks of nuts and seeds in the crust but make sure the dates are blended throughout.

Filling:

Use your favorite apples (about 4 to 6 fresh apples depending on the size of the apples and the size of your pie dish) mixed evenly with dried apples (about 2 large handfuls), half fresh and half dried. Let your food processor grind them up nicely. Fill your pie crust with the end product, and you have a delicious AND nutritious dessert! You can use thinly sliced apples to garnish your pie. I suggest refrigerating for at least 10 to 15 minutes before serving to help the ingredients bind together. You can also use different fillings like sliced bananas and/or mangos instead of apples for a raw tropical pie.

This is a very short list of the possibilities that exist for you. I encourage you to experiment for yourself and get creative.

SUMMARY

················ ✦ ✦ ················

HEALTH IS NOT A BUSINESS

After reading a first draft of this work an acquaintance asked me, "Why should I listen to you?" "You shouldn't," I told him. You shouldn't listen to me or be obedient to ANY one (health professional, nutritionist, association, society) unless **you know** their methods have truly helped others and they have no motive other than to aid you. Take this tremendous opportunity to do one of the rarest things a human being can do—THINK FOR YOURSELF. Oh, the trouble we could avoid and the beauty we could touch if we were practiced at this rare art of self-reliance and if we would stop assuming that only a credentialed person can have something of value to say and that those without them are not worth a listen. It is a common practice to at-tack the messenger if the message is not what we expect or want to hear, especially if the message is a threat to business. Assess what you have been presented here; if it seems reasonable, fairly and thoroughly apply the advice to yourself and see if things do not get better. You can have your own empirical evidence, be your own scientist, and work in the most incredible laboratory ever invented, your body.

Concerning "credentials," I have one question for you. Who is in charge of the "health" care system in this country? The answer is the heavily credentialed American Medical Association is in charge. If credentials equal wisdom and competence, why is it that our country is in such a disease-ridden state and so rapidly on the decline with more obese people than any other country in the world, with more deaths from cancer and heart disease than ever before, and with the most heavily drugged child population mankind has ever known? History has proven time and again that blind faith in our leaders is a disastrous practice.

I hope I have presented you with a logical and sound model for healthy living and a new perspective on disease and health. My wish is that something in you is thinking *this makes sense*. I can assure you that I have personally seen hundreds of sick and dying individuals return themselves to health through this natural means.

You might also want to consider the fact that I am not selling you anything. There are no products to buy, no powders, no special formulas or pills, no *new age program*, and no way for me to profit from your heeding these suggestions and abiding by Natural Laws.

Any endeavor that grants precious rewards does require great discipline and effort. I am quite aware of what a transformation this way of abiding by Nature's Laws is for our thinking and living, especially considering our present circumstance. I am also conscious of the resistance that may result when you realize the "sacrifices" that you must endure. To some of you it may seem to be a difficult if not impossible way of life. You must remember and realize that **all of your present habits, good or bad, have been learned and can be unlearned.** ***Do not underestimate what you are capable of doing***.

Our brains have been wired, mostly unconsciously, in a certain way to which we have grown accustomed, heavily influenced by our culture, parents, and immediate surroundings. In his book *Your Maximum Mind,* Dr. Herbert Benson of the Harvard Medical School describes how this mind organization occurs:

> *Over the years you develop 'circuits' and 'channels' of thought in your brain. These are physical pathways, which control the way you think, the way you act, and often the way you feel. Many times these pathways become so fixed that they turn into what I call 'wiring.' In other words the circuits or channels become so deeply ingrained that it seems almost impossible to transform them.*

There are approximately 100 billion nerve cells in the brain, and each of these communicates with the others through connections called synapses. The total number of possible connections is 25,000,000,000,000,000,000,000,000,000,000,000, Dr. Benson estimates. Put another way, if you were to stack sheets of typing paper with each sheet representing a neuron connection, the resulting pile would be approximately 16 billion light years high, extending beyond the limits of the known universe.

Robert Ornstein MD, another renowned brain researcher from the University of California, claims that the number of possible connections in the brain is greater than the number of atoms in the universe.

It seems, according to these scientists, that the possibility for our brains making new connections is unlimited. Please do not sell yourself short by thinking that you are your past. You are MUCH greater than you know.

I can only TELL you what a wonderful gift it is to live according to Natural Laws and make you aware of the magnificent benefits this way of life affords me and the growing number of those who are catching on to this shining way of life. I can also tell you of the hundreds of people who have been left for dead by today's *health experts* who are now leading disease-free, vigorous lives with great confidence in their physical abilities without worry that their previous conditions will return. I also can tell you of the guaranteed success of those looking to lose weight as well as those once afflicted with asthma, diabetes, herpes, AIDS, cancer, etc., who are now living drug free, asymptomatic, healthy lives.

You must EXPERIENCE the increased energy, loss of fat, glowing skin, mental alertness, and overall vitality this raw food regimen brings with it in order to UNDER-STAND. It is impossible for you to accurately imagine the benefits, and to try to do so is a big mistake.

> *The only source of knowledge is experience.*
> —Albert Einstein

The idea that you will be living a life of deprivation and have to give up certain foods is an illusion equivalent to telling a prisoner he should stay in his rat-infested jail cell because he will miss the wildlife if he were to walk out. Eventually you will not be missing anything, and you will be thrilled about your new way of life. It may take some time, but if you make sincere efforts toward this transition, the rewards to be experienced are beyond your imagination.

As far as the idea of deprivation and being *bored* by the natural regime, I can assure you that there are simply no serious raw foodists complaining of boredom. After a while your body will reestablish its natural cravings. This transition to health may take a year or two. It makes sense to consider the time your body has spent on the *normal* toxic diet and realize that weaning yourself off the addictive foods and additives requires some work. Those who have made a sincere and lasting effort have nothing but praise and stories of delightful transformation. I can remember on many occasions complaining that there was *nothing to eat* when I was on the SAD diet. Of course, being bored about what to eat has nothing to do with lack of food choices; it is simply indicative of the deranged attitude we have toward food.

Eating with the idea of entertaining ourselves creates food addiction and will lead to an unending passion quest that can never be satisfied.

It is quite an experience to taste a fruit the way it was meant to be tasted with re-awakened, re-sensitized taste buds. It is a whole other sense of wonder to have your body operating the way in which it was intended with improved digestion, vision, and hearing, something very few human beings ever experience.

COMFORT FOODS ARE FOODS THAT MAKE YOU THE MOST UN- COMFORTABLE.

Making the transition may be a challenge, but I assure you there is nothing boring about living according to your true nature; in fact it may be the most exciting thing you have ever experienced. Making this transition is the equivalent of running your car in first gear for years and all of a sudden discovering that there are three other gears.

You will also save a considerable amount of money by staying healthy, avoiding regular trips to the doctor, and having no need to buy any type of remedial product, prescription, or over-the-counter drugs. If you or a family member becomes ill, there will be no question of how to deal with it.

It is also important to realize that there is an entire world of raw food preparation available to you. There are many raw food preparation books on the market these days. I am pleased to see that the idea of raw eating is catching on. Unfortunately many of these preparation manuals have included heavily spiced, processed and irritating menus. It would be best to avoid using molasses, refined sugars, onions, garlic, honey, table or sea salt, pepper, and any processed food or liquid.

> *Excessive care of the body, is most inimical to the practice of virtue.*
>
> —Plato

If you are seriously ill or have been suffering from chronic health problems for years, a resolute and stringent discipline may be required for your recovery. An immediate and complete cessation of any foods and toxins that do not belong in the body and an adherence to Natural Laws may make the difference between life and death. In such cases, strict compliance to proper feeding and care of the body is paramount.

If you are not in such a debilitated physical condition, it would behoove you to recognize the difficulty of the task at hand and to take a reasonable approach to making this life-changing transition. There are some people who come upon this knowledge and immediately take it upon themselves to give up all their unnatural feeding habits. This type of complete and determined effort is rare under normal circumstances. Assessing and measuring the difficulties you may incur is a wise move, especially when there are others in your household. Way too often families are disrupted and irreparably upset because of a reformed individual that insists, "everyone must change now that I have." This is a sort of violence that can be more disease-producing than a drug-laden steak.

Remember that eating right is a major factor in the quality of our health, but it is not the most important one. It may be more important to keep the peace in your home rather than fighting to change everybody now that you are ready to change. I suggest if these ideas of living resonate in you and you have the interest and inclination to begin to live according to Nature's Laws, it is better if you do it for yourself at first without imposing your will on your friends or family. There is nothing more inviting than the power of example. It is possible that others will also see the benefits of this way of life.

Certainly you can present these ideas to your family members and loved ones. You can SUGGEST that they read this book. If they are resistant, do both yourself and them a favor and LEAVE THEM ALONE.

It is extremely frustrating to see family members and loved ones involved in daily poisoning acts and thoughtless, ravaging "treatments" that you know are absurd and dangerous. However, it is equally absurd to try to change somebody who does not want to change. One of the most difficult lessons I have learned and continue to learn is that some people would rather die horrible deaths than change. This is a fact that is sometimes hard to swallow but is evident throughout our society. There is not one adult in the civilized world that does not know that smoking causes cancer and death, yet millions of people continue to engage in this activity and spend their money to kill themselves.

DO NOT TRY TO CHANGE OTHERS.

I once saw a man who, after thirty years of smoking, had to have a major throat surgery for the cancer that had invaded his esophagus and vocal cords. After the operation, he had to be fed through a plastic tube inserted in his neck. Now devoid of vocal chords and a large part of his neck, unable to speak or eat, this man insisted on his *smoking pleasure* and would put a lit cigarette into the tube and inhale. This is a testimony to the willfulness and obdurate nature of human beings disinterested in change.

Just because what you are proposing has been tried, tested, true, and effective, not everybody wants to hear it. In fact, MOST people do not want to hear it. Some of the greatest teachers ever to walk this planet were mocked, ostracized, persecuted, and put to death because of the truthful message they imparted. Do not waste your energies trying to force a change in others.

Remember: we live in an insane world—any moves or efforts toward sanity will absolutely guarantee accusations and charges of insanity from the insane. Do not put yourself in harm's way by making an issue of your new way of living. Most people do not want to hear it, and you are doing yourself damage by bringing it up to the disinterested.

OBSESSIVE BEHAVIOR

Most people do not take any time to examine their eating habits or consider the consequences of just eating like everybody else. Obviously there is a price to pay for this lack of responsibility. On the other end of the spectrum, there are those who become obsessive about their eating choices and unreasonable when it comes to their physical maintenance. This type of compulsion and rigid neurotic behavior is disease-producing in and of itself and makes for a very unpleasant person.

Enthusiasm and excitement are imminent as you learn about and experience the effects of eating well and caring for the body. I certainly encourage you to share your joy and enthusiasm with those who are interested, but I only can warn you about the perils of trying to change others who are disinterested or who are about becoming self-righteous.

Unfortunately there are those who will take the idea of nutrition WAY too far and make it the only focus in their life.

> *Truth is our element of life; yet if a man fasten his attention on a single aspect of truth and apply himself to that alone for a long time, the truth becomes distorted and not itself but falsehood.*

> —Emerson

Balance is lost by obsessive and exaggerated attention devoted to nutrition; It is one thing to be dedicated and disciplined about the care of your body; it is another thing to be overly concerned and neurotic about it. A life unbalanced is painful and disease-producing. My suggestion is that you assess your personal condition and your lifestyle, consider exactly what you would like to achieve in terms of improving your health, make some specific goals, do your best to achieve them, and let go of the result. However, if you are in physical pain and gravely ill, I suggest an intense level of commitment. Do not forget to keep a sense of humor about yourself and enjoy the process.

There are those who use their eating habits as a means to express their anger, avoid others, feel superior, and distract themselves from the real issues in their lives by compulsively talking and thinking about eating. I highly suggest you avoid this type of behavior. If you find yourself constantly defending yourself and arguing with others you can bet that you are doing more harm than good. It is fairly easy to tell who is interested in these ideas and who is not. Learn to be diplomatic and to disengage those that want to argue and fight and relish those who have a sincere interest in improving their health.

Remember that there is nothing more important to your well being than the contents of your heart and mind. If you are constantly tense, anxiety-ridden, angry, resentful, and worried, your chances of achieving health are negligible. We are spiritual beings in a physical body; act accordingly and feed your spirit. Starting your day with a sitting meditation is a most beneficial practice. Keeping a daily journal will allow your mind to slow down, give you the ability to assess just what it is that may be bothering you, and give you a clear opportunity to express yourself. Reading the works of great minds, many whom have been quoted in this book, will provide you with constant inspiration to reach above and beyond the daily quagmire of mechanical thinking and unconscious behavior so prevalent in today's world. Of course, eating properly will be a tremendous aid to your spiritual growth, as a finely tuned body increases one's receptivity to higher ideas.

Exercise is essential to our well being, and going without a regular physical regime is harmful to your body. A gentle discipline is necessary. Do not count activity such as walking to work or cleaning the house as exercise. Spend at least fifteen to twenty minutes a day doing some type of disciplined exercise where there is no distraction. Yoga, rebounding, bike riding, fast walking, swimming, or resistance training including calisthenics or weight training are all very effective disciplines that can be done in your home. Wherever there is a floor and gravity you can train. Do not waste your energy making excuses why you cannot exercise. **If you do not have twenty minutes a day to spend on yourself, your lifestyle must change.**

Make sure you leave some time, even if it is only a half an hour a week (although I do suggest more), to do some kind of activity that you enjoy such as playing a musical instrument, sculpting, dancing, singing, painting, or drawing. These artistic endeavors can also be tremendous boon to your well being.

One of the most common situations I come across when counseling sickly individuals is their tendency to make themselves SO busy that they have *legitimate excuses* for not taking proper care of themselves. **Staying busy is a disease in and of itself that is sure to manifest itself physically.** The desperation to constantly be on the run or on the phone or DOING something is evidence of great emotional turmoil that is being ignored and, even worse, denied. Most of the world is doing this in some form or another, and this staying overly busy is the cause of great physical, mental, and emotional anguish.

We are human beings, not human doings. Most people are frightened of a quiet moment because that would mean facing themselves. So we have invented endless arrays of distractions to take the attention off what really needs attention. Eating is a prime distraction along with over working, smoking, drinking, television, talking, focusing on others, creating or involving ourselves in some type of human conflict or emergency.

Our problems gain size, strength, and speed with each evasion. The more we run from our problems, the more they show up in our lives. And the more they show up in our lives, the more we need to distract ourselves—a truly vicious cycle. The opposite is thankfully true. If you are willing to stand and face the difficulties in your life, those difficulties will LOSE power and strength, and YOU will gain power and strength.

LIVING IN THE DARK IS DANGEROUS.

Then you will no longer be a constant slave to your obsessive behaviors and avoidances, and gain some balance in your life. The "freedom" that most people talk about is an insatiable never-ending sensual slavery. The only true freedom that exists lies in obedience to higher laws.

Just because most of the world is living in the dark and you have grown accustomed to the world's habitual pains and sufferings does not mean you must go on smashing into the furniture or falling down and injuring yourself. *There is A WAY OUT.* You have a choice. **Every second that passes you make a choice whether to think in your old familiar ways or to try something different.** If you do what you have always done, you get what you have always gotten. A good definition of insanity is doing the same thing but expecting a different result. Allowing yourself to be formed and molded by a society gone mad is a guarantee that YOU will also be mad.

If these ideas make sense to you and you wish to implement this program, I would suggest that you **make a consistent and regular study of this book.** It is one thing to read this once and think it makes sense; it is another thing to summon up the necessary energy and desire to go against years of mis-education and a world gone mad. Do not underestimate the force of belief. The ideas in this book are a tremendous threat to the status quo, and implementing these ideas requires great confidence and certainty.

Making these conscious choices to change your eating habits is a sign that you no longer want to live the way most people do. You are affirming that you will no longer succumb to your addictive and destructive behaviors in the physical world. These efforts, combined with the re-awakening of the body, increase the receptivity of your being which allows for a greater possibility for inner transformation and your overall wellness.

ABOUT THE AUTHOR

Matthew Grace, diagnosed with Multiple Sclerosis and Spinal Chord Degeneration, was unable to stand or move his legs. Gripped by severe numbness and fatigue, he was crippled and given little hope for any recovery and no chance to walk again. Grace is now back on his feet. For years he has been sharing his extraordinary recovery experience with riveted audiences. Refusing ALL conventional treatments and working "from the inside out," this man, doomed by modern medicine, found his way back to health. His story is a remarkable tale of self-discovery and physical transformation.

A former standout amateur boxer, fitness expert, and author, his services and expertise have been sought out by many, including some of our top celebrities. The president and founder of the Coalition for Health Re-Education, Grace has helped hundreds of people diagnosed with incurable disease re-gain their health.

He has appeared on *Prime Time Live* with Diane Sawyer and *Good Day New York*, hosted a New York-based cable television program for seven years, and appeared on numerous radio programs.

For many years this man has been inspiring audiences with his remarkable story; his mission, "to let people know there is A WAY OUT, no matter what you are facing," is complimented by his insightful, philosophical and often humorous delivery.